60 WAYS

TO LOWER YOUR

CHOLESTEROL

ROBERT D. LESSLIE, MD

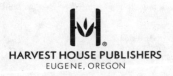

HARVEST HOUSE PUBLISHERS
EUGENE, OREGON

Cover by Koechel Peterson & Associates, Minneapolis, Minnesota

This book is not intended to take the place of sound professional medical advice. Neither the author nor the publisher assumes any liability for possible adverse consequences as a result of the information contained herein.

Unless otherwise noted, the stories in this book are fictitious accounts, used for illustration purposes only. Although based on the author's experiences, they are not meant to refer to any person, living or dead.

60 WAYS TO LOWER YOUR CHOLESTEROL
Copyright © 2015 by Robert D. Lesslie, MD
Published by Harvest House Publishers
Eugene, Oregon 97402
www.harvesthousepublishers.com

Library of Congress Cataloging-in-Publication Data
Lesslie, Robert D., 1951-
60 ways to lower your cholesterol / Robert D. Lesslie, MD.
    pages cm
title: Sixty ways to lower your cholesterol
ISBN 978-0-7369-6325-1 (pbk.)
ISBN 978-0-7369-6326-8 (eBook)
1. Hypercholesteremia—Popular works. 2. Hypercholesteremia–Treatment—Popular works. I. Title. II. Title: Sixty ways to lower your cholesterol.
RC632.H83L47 2015
616.3'997—dc23

                                                    2014045692

Printed in the United States of America

          15 16 17 18 19 20 21 22 23 / VP-JH / 10 9 8 7 6 5 4 3 2 1

Dedication

As a bagpiper, I quickly learned you can't teach yourself how to play this unique and complicated instrument. You need an instructor. And I have learned something else. The relationship becomes much more than that of teacher/student. A special bond develops, something deep and spiritual. The teacher imparts a gift, a piece of himself, and that piece abides forever with the student.

If you are fortunate, the same becomes true of the relationship between a writer and his editor. It has become true for me. This book, along with my deepest and abiding gratitude, is dedicated to *my* editor, Paul Gossard.

> *"You have not lived*
> *until you have done something for someone*
> *who can never repay you."*
>
> ANONYMOUS

Contents

Welcome!

"Say Doc, can you help me live a shorter life and make my health a little worse?"

You're right. In almost forty years of practicing medicine, I've never been asked that question. Just the opposite. Who doesn't want to enjoy the best health possible?

By God's design we are complex creatures, and our well-being is dependent on caring for our spiritual, emotional, and physical health. We can't afford to neglect any of these. In this book we will be focusing on the *physical* element and how to take the necessary steps to ensure that this part of our health is as good as it can be.

If you're reading these words, you must be at least a little interested in, or maybe even concerned about, one aspect of this well-being—your cholesterol level. So we start off with something in common. And if your level is abnormal—as is mine—and you have a family history of heart disease—as do I—we have something even more in common.

This is important stuff, especially when it comes to living as well as we can for as long as we can. Elevated cholesterol (and other lipids) is a known risk factor for heart disease and other serious health problems. But it's sneaky. As with high blood pressure, it creeps up on you with no obvious warning signals until a lot of damage has been done. The good news is there's something we can do about it. And the better news is it's not going to be difficult.

In the following pages, you'll meet Lisa and Dave Jernigan, a couple who may be very similar to you or someone you know. This book is about their journey as we work together to define and control their cholesterol problems. It *will* be a journey, filled with setbacks, confusion, misinformation, disappointments, but most importantly—small and large victories.

Here you'll find everything you need to understand and manage your own lipid levels, improve your overall health, and begin your unique journey. You'll find the bare bones information necessary to get you started. For those who want a more technical approach as to how all this fits together, you'll find plenty of sections titled "Give Me the Details, Doc."

Although we will be focusing on our physical health, it's impossible to separate this or anything else from our spiritual lives. What won't be lost on us as we work through all of this is the complexity and interrelatedness of our bodies. Indeed, we are "fearfully and wonderfully made" (Psalm 139:14).

This is a good time to introduce you to Lisa and Dave.

1

We've Got Work to Do

Wendy plopped two patient charts in front of me.

"The Jernigans are in room 2. I just checked their vital signs, and all that looks good. I put their lab reports in their files."

She took a few steps toward the nurses' office, stopped, and turned to face me. "And good luck with *Mr.* Jernigan."

I shook my head but didn't look up. I understood.

Dave Jernigan was a forty-six-year-old college professor of US history. Steeped in the musty tomes of our founding fathers, his preoccupation with his teaching had led to a woeful neglect of his own well-being.

"Haven't been to a doctor in twenty years," he had proudly declared last week in our office. His wife had finally hounded him long enough to bring him in for an examination and routine blood work.

"Don't really see the point of this, Doctor," he said. "I feel fine. Could stand to lose a few pounds, I suppose, but other than that, I'm in great shape."

Lisa Jernigan was a year younger than her husband and had taught high school algebra and calculus for almost two decades. She had taught two of our children, and I knew her to be tough, analytical, and dedicated to her students. While Dave would be champing at the bit to get out of the office, Lisa would have a lot of questions, especially after I shared their lab reports with them.

I closed the door of room 2 behind me. Lisa looked up from where she was sitting and smiled.

"Good morning, Robert," she said. "I hope you've got some good news for us."

Dave sat on the exam table, his hands under his thighs. Our eyes met, and he nodded and then gazed back down at the floor.

"In fact, I *do* have good news." I pulled the remaining chair out from the wall and sat down. "For the most part."

"The most part?"

"Let's start with your lab report, Lisa. As we discussed last week, your blood pressure is fine—115 over 78—and your EKG is completely normal." I flipped through the top couple of pages of her file, looking for the sheet of lab numbers. "Everything here looks good—your hemoglobin, blood sugar, liver studies. And your thyroid study continues to be good."

She smiled and nodded. She had a strong family history of hypothyroidism, including her mother and two sisters. Thus far, she had been spared.

"The only thing that's out of line is your triglyceride level. The upper limit is 150, and this time yours is 278. It's been gradually creeping up the past few years, but this is the highest it's been."

"I've been taking fish oil every day," Lisa said. "I thought that was supposed to help. What about my cholesterol level?"

"It's fine—175. And your good cholesterol is where it's supposed to be, as is your LDL, the bad cholesterol."

"Well, at least *that's* a good thing." She sighed and folded her hands in her lap. "So what now? How do we get that number down? To 150, isn't that what you said?"

"That's right. We'll want to get your triglycerides back to normal, and there are several ways we can do that."

"Good to know. Now what about Dave? Is everything okay with his labs?"

I closed Lisa's chart and tossed it onto the exam table, then opened Dave's chart and thumbed through several forms and reports. "Your blood pressure was okay, Dave—borderline at 132 over 86. We'll keep an eye on that. But your urine, EKG, and chest X-ray are all normal. Just like your wife, all of your labs look great until we get to your lipids."

"My what?"

"Your lipids, honey," Lisa said. "Your cholesterol—the good and the bad—and your triglycerides. Those are your lipids, aren't they, Robert?"

"That's right. The good news, Dave, is your triglyceride level is normal—138. But your total cholesterol is 289 and your LDL is 160."

Lisa glanced at her husband and then back to me. "Those are dangerous numbers, aren't they?"

"They're high but not dangerous. Not unless we don't do anything about them."

"Where should those numbers be?" Lisa asked. "What would be good?"

"As far as the cholesterol, we want to see that number below 200. With the LDL, a lot of people think it's okay at 120, but my goal would be 100 or less. Especially considering your..."

I hesitated just long enough for Lisa to finish my sentence. "Especially considering Dave's family history."

"That's right. We've got work to do. Dave, with your family history, we need to be a little more—"

"Listen, Doc, what's the big deal?"

What *Is* the Big Deal?

Thomas Skelton, a publican, forty-seven years of age, being rather lusty, subject to frequent colds, attended with coughs, hoarseness, and a discharge of matter from the lungs or throat, but otherwise enjoying a good state of health, was attacked with a violent cold, together with a difficulty of breathing, and applied to Mr. Wilson, apothecary, who took twelve ounces of blood from his arm, which relieved him greatly. He had taken some bread and butter, with some tea, without milk, about four hours before he was bled. The blood coagulated firmly, and the serum which separated, was of a white colour, with a yellowish tinge, appearing like the colour of cream; upon the top of this floated a white scum, like another cream.

More than two hundred years ago, John Hunter, an English physician, knew something was up when he described this blood specimen of one of his patients. That "white scum" was almost certainly a layer of cholesterol and fat floating in Thomas Skelton's blood.

This condition has been causing problems for a long time, and was causing a problem now for Dave Jernigan. My challenge was to get his attention and convince him this needed to be fixed. Fortunately, that fix wouldn't involve any bloodletting.

"Okay, Dave, let's talk about your two boys." Lisa and Dave had twin twenty-year-old sons, Adam and Seth.

Dave's head snapped up. "What do they have to do with my health problems?"

"I think Robert is trying to make the point that you need to be around for the boys," Lisa said, "when they graduate from Clemson, get married, have children."

"And someday grandchildren," I added. "That's a whole new ballgame, Dave, and you don't want to miss any of it. My job is to give you the best possible chance to be there."

"Robert, you and I both know there are no guarantees," Dave said. "Our days are numbered, and all that. I'm not convinced there's much I can do to..." His head slumped and he rubbed his hands together.

"How old were you when your father died?"

He looked up at me, his face flushed. "Ten, almost eleven." His voice was quiet. "And yes, I miss him and wish he was still around. Not just for me, but for Adam and Seth."

The room was silent for a moment, then Dave straightened himself and looked directly at me. "But his heart attack, it was a family thing. He was only thirty-eight when he died, and his father and my two brothers all died young. All of them had heart attacks. What makes you think I can avoid that? None of them smoked, and I don't either. I don't know about their blood pressures."

"But they all had trouble with their cholesterol," Lisa said. "Or at least your brothers did."

"And we know you don't have diabetes," I added. "Those are all big risk factors when it comes to heart disease and strokes, and you've got them under control. We can't change your genes, but we *can* do something about your cholesterol. The good thing is, you know your numbers. You gotta know your numbers."

You Gotta Know Your Numbers

Clyde Anderson

The ER, Tuesday, 2:30 p.m.

"Dr. Lesslie, I need you to see the man in room 4."

Lori Davidson was our triage nurse this afternoon, and she wore a worried look. She handed the patient's clipboard to me and nodded toward the curtained room.

"He just doesn't look right. Pale, almost pasty, and his blood pressure is a little low. His wife is in there with him and can give you a good history. He seems a little confused. There's no one in triage right now, so I'd be glad to help."

"Great," I said, glancing down at the record. "Let's go."

Clyde Anderson
58-year-old male
Upper abdominal pain
Pulse 106, BP 100/60, temp 100.6

I closed the curtain behind us and stepped over to the stretcher. Clyde Anderson was a large man, probably over six-two and two hundred and fifty pounds. He was lying on the bed with his eyes closed, arms folded across his chest. Lori was right—he was pale. No, he was pasty.

His wife was standing at the head of the stretcher and turned to us.

"I'm Rosemary—Rosemary Anderson." Her brow was furrowed, and she glanced back and forth from me to her husband. "He's been sick for a couple of days, but really bad the past twenty-four hours or so."

"Any medical problems that you know of?"

Rosemary chuckled but without any mirth. "How would we know? He hasn't been to the doctor in more than ten years. Not until two days ago when I finally convinced him to go see my family physician. That's when I knew he was sick and in pain. Otherwise, he'd still be at home."

I looked at the record again and saw the name of their doctor.

"What did Dr. Ballard think was going on?"

My hand was now on Clyde's abdomen, gently examining for any signs of tenderness or rigidity. He moaned quietly but didn't move.

"He wasn't as sick then as he is now. Dr. Ballard looked at him and thought it might be bad indigestion or something called reflux, I think. He prescribed some medication—Prevacid—and Clyde's been taking it like he's supposed to, but it's not helping. He's just getting worse."

"You want the lab?" Lori whispered in my ear.

"Yeah, and let's get an IV of normal saline started."

I turned back to Rosemary. "Has Clyde had any surgery? Any gall-bladder problems or a stomach ulcer?"

"No, he's always been in good health. No surgery and no medicines—not until we started this Prevacid."

"Any blood pressure problems?" It was low right now, especially for his size, and that worried me.

"Like I said, how would we know? He hasn't been to a doctor in more than ten years, maybe more."

"So you wouldn't know about any diabetes or heart trouble or anything like that?"

She shook her head and looked down at her husband. "No idea."

A few minutes later, the lab tech was in the room, filling a half-dozen glass vials with blood. Without looking up or saying a word, she handed me a red-stoppered tube.

"What do you—" I glanced down at the vial and understood. The bottom of the tube was filled with bright-red blood, but the top third was nothing but a whitish cream. Fat. I had never seen anything like it.

When the initial labs were returned, we had our diagnosis. Pancreatitis. Clyde's lipase and amylase levels were sky-high. It took a while longer for his lipids to be reported, and it was worse than I imagined. His cholesterol was elevated at 250, but his triglyceride level—the amount of fat in his blood—was over 2,000. That was astronomical, and was causing his pancreatitis.

Clyde Anderson's ticket had been punched. He was on a journey that neither he nor his wife could have imagined just a few days earlier.

Over the next few hours, his blood pressure started to fall. We were giving him IV fluids and doing everything we could to support him. One of the GI specialists was admitting him to the ICU and had called in an internist, Jack Flanders, to help.

It was Jack who came to the ER to tell me about Clyde's abdominal CT scan.

"I don't think I've ever seen anything like it, Robert. He's already leaking fluid into his peritoneal space. And his pancreas—it's disintegrating right in front of our eyes—auto-digesting itself. His calcium level is way out of whack and so are his electrolytes. He's had three units of blood, and we still can't get his blood pressure stabilized."

Flanders shook his head. "I'm headed back to the ICU and will give you a call if something changes."

The next morning, we learned Clyde had been helicoptered to Duke. His condition had continued to deteriorate, and Jack Flanders and the GI specialist had reached out to some friends at the Duke Medical Center— experts in dealing with diseases of the pancreas. Clyde was still on that journey—that train ride—and there was no getting off.

A week passed, and Lori and I stood at the nurses' station.

"Have you heard anything about Mr. Anderson?" she asked, rummaging in her pocket and pulling out a scrap of paper.

"No, I haven't. I wonder if—"

"Rosemary Anderson gave me her cell number." She unfolded the note and reached for the telephone on the counter. "I'll give her a call and see how he's doing."

Lori dialed the number and waited.

"Mrs. Anderson, this is Lori Davidson at the hospital in Rock Hill. I was calling to check on your husband."

She listened intently for a moment, her head nodding from time to time. Then she looked up at me with wide eyes and shook her head.

Clyde was gone.

4

Give Me the Details, Doc

What's the Risk?

We've known for a while about the problems with abnormal blood lipids—various cholesterols and fats—collectively known as hyperlipidemia. It's only been over the past few decades that our knowledge has been refined and we truly understand the magnitude of the harm these conditions can cause.

Hyperlipidemias can significantly increase the risk of a wide range of maladies:

- cardiovascular diseases of the blood vessels supplying the heart, brain, arms, and legs
- chest pain (angina), heart attacks, heart failure, strokes, and sudden death
- aortic atherosclerosis and thoracic or abdominal aortic aneurysms
- inflammation of the pancreas (pancreatitis)

But what's the risk here, and what does it mean for you and me? As of this writing, cardiovascular disease, heart disease, and stroke account for most of the deaths each year in the United States and in other developed countries. There are multiple risk factors for these problems, of which hyperlipidemia continues to be one of the leading. For those of you interested in figures, the Centers for Disease Control (CDC) maintains a public website at CDC.gov. The most recent ranking of causes of death in the US are:

1. heart disease

2. cancer

3. COPD (emphysema and chronic bronchitis)

4. stroke

5. accidents

Of these, heart disease and cancer cause almost half the annual deaths in this country.

These are impressive statistics, but they relate only to the number of deaths caused by these diseases. These disorders also take a significant toll on those who live with them, as well as on their loved ones and caregivers. A stroke radically changes things for all involved, and a heart attack can drastically alter a person's quality of life.

The silver lining here is that these significant problems are largely preventable. Most of us know the risk factors for heart disease and stroke: increasing age, male gender, smoking, hypertension, diabetes, obesity, heredity, and elevated cholesterol. Whereas your gender and genetic makeup have been determined, and slowing or reversing the aging process has eluded our best efforts, there are elements here that can be modified. And by modifying them, we can prevent a lot of premature deaths and needless suffering.

But that modifying process doesn't just happen. It requires real effort, discipline, and determination. Most importantly, it requires the knowledge that we have an actual problem. It is frequently said, and rightly so, that high blood pressure is a silent killer. Unannounced, it hammers away at your heart and brain and kidneys without you knowing it—until something bad happens.

The same can be said about elevated cholesterol and blood fats. The arteries of our bodies slowly become occluded by yellowish, greasy plaques, gradually increasing in size until they reach a critical mass. By the time we develop symptoms, there's a big problem. Those symptoms can be sudden, such as a stroke or sudden death. Or they can begin slowly, as with the calf and leg pains associated with claudication—lack of blood flow to these muscles due to clogged arteries. This is the same process that causes angina—lack of blood flow to our heart muscle—and starts with pain with exercise and exertion. Again, once this happens, something major is going on.

Another thing that makes all of this a big deal is how early the process starts. Usually, we don't develop symptoms from elevated lipids and atherosclerosis ("hardening of the arteries") until we reach our fifties or sixties. But those yellowish deposits start long before that—sometimes as early as in our teenage years. We know that many, if not most, young male soldiers whose lives were ended in their twenties already have clear evidence of this process in their major arteries. This especially happens in the aorta, but it is also present in the coronary arteries of the heart.

So this is a big deal. The disease starts early, worsens gradually and silently, affects most of us, and involves critical organs and body systems. And it can be prevented. If already started, it can be managed—maybe even reversed.

But you have to know about it. And you have to know your numbers and what to do with them.

Okay, I Get It

"Alright, Doc, you got my attention. So, tell me what my numbers are again and what they need to be. I wasn't listening the first time."

Dave was being honest, and that was progress. I opened his chart and flipped to the lab report.

"Your total cholesterol is 289. That number needs to be below 200 [see chapter 14 for detailed information about cholesterol]. And your LDL, the bad cholesterol, is 160. That needs to be below 100 [see chapter 24]."

"Wait a minute, isn't there a *good* cholesterol?" Dave said. "What about that?"

"You're right. There *is* a good cholesterol—your HDL—and that number is borderline. It needs to be above 40, and yours is 39. That's not too bad, but the higher the better [see chapter 18]."

"What would be a good number, Dr. Lesslie?" Lisa asked.

"Somewhere in the 50s would be fine. If we can get it into the 60s or 70s, that would be great. But right now, it's okay. We need to focus on Dave's LDL. That's the one that concerns me."

"And his triglycerides?" Lisa said. "You said they were normal, didn't you?"

My finger swept the lab sheet. "Yes, that's fine. It needs to be below 150, and Dave's at 138 [see chapter 36]."

"Well, at least there's *some* good news," Dave said with a huff.

"There's a lot of good news here, Dave. It's good that we know your numbers now, and it's good that we can do something about it."

"And about my triglycerides too," Lisa said. "We can work on this together."

Dave folded his arms across his chest, took a deep breath, and sighed. "Alright, where do we start? But keep this in mind, Dr. Lesslie—I don't want to be on a pill for the rest of my life."

"There are a lot of things to do before we get to that point," I said. "Let's take a look at those and see how things go."

Getting Started

Each of us is different, with our unique and peculiar circumstances and quirks. That's a good thing. We don't all weigh the same. Some of us are tall and some are short. Some of us have "good genes," while others seem to be genetically challenged with family histories loaded with diabetes, heart trouble, and cancer. And to make matters even worse, some folks who don't live in the South speak with strange accents.

It is this uniqueness, this variability that makes the practice of medicine challenging and, at the same time, very rewarding. One size doesn't fit everyone. And while we all put our pants on one leg at a time, those pants are different colors, different sizes, and different styles.

So, how do we get started when it comes to managing problems with our cholesterol and other lipids? Fortunately, it all begins with one word: *lifestyle.* That's where we're going to start. We're going to take a look at the things we do that impact our health, and the things we don't do that might help us.

The first big area we need to focus on is our *diet*—what we put into our bodies. We are in fact what we eat. That can sometimes be pretty scary. One of the amazing things about our body is its ability to make do with what we feed it. There is a certain amount of leeway when it comes to extracting the correct balance of proteins, carbohydrates, and fats from our GI tract. Our diets don't have to be perfect to give us what we need. But there is a limit.

Then there's our liver—the most efficient detoxifier on this planet. It hums along, extracting poisons from our bloodstream, chemically altering them just enough to allow for their excretion through our intestines. But again, there's a limit. A good example of this would be our old friend EtOH—*ethyl alcohol*. We can handle a certain amount of this chemical, but when that limit is exceeded, the cells in our liver start shutting down, and we're in trouble.

So it's all about balance. And that's where lifestyle comes into play. Our lives need to be in balance, beginning with what we eat and drink. We'll take a look at the multitude of diets and fads currently in vogue, and what makes the most sense for the most people.

Next up will be *exercise*. We'll consider why this is so important, what kinds of exercise are the most efficient, and what dangers lie in store for those of us who neglect this important part of our well-being. There's good news here as well. Mounting evidence clearly demonstrates we don't have to run marathons or compete in triathlons to have a big impact on our health. Simple and painless activities are all that's required, and no matter what your age or physical condition, there's something for everyone.

One of the benefits of regular and adequate exercise is the reduction of *stress*. What, you may ask, does stress have to do with a balanced lifestyle? A bunch, it seems. We live in an anxious, stressed-out culture. Just look around you. People rushing here and there—deadlines to meet, meetings to attend, projects to complete. Hmm…sounds a little too familiar.

But all of this stress takes a toll on our health. Anxiety is clearly associated with the development of heart disease, diabetes, hypertension, and other significant problems. We need to identify the stressors in our lives and eliminate them, when possible. Again, it's all about balance. A little stress is healthy for us. It's when it overpowers us that things start breaking down.

One of those things that break down is our *sleep*. This is another very important part of our well-being and hinges on a healthy lifestyle. Inadequate sleep is a factor in the development of a lot of serious complications, including heart disease as well as diabetes and high blood pressure. We're going to explore simple ways to improve our sleep patterns, learn when it's important to undergo professional testing, and consider effective treatments when we have a real problem.

Sleep and cholesterol? Yep, that's right. It all ties together—intricately interwoven. One aspect of our health impacts another and another and another. It's all about balance.

Our individual lifestyles embrace much more than what we've talked about so far, including our close and significant relationships, our spiritual health, even our dreams and aspirations.

But we've got plenty to work with thus far, so let's get going.

7

Give Me the Details, Doc

What Exactly Are We Talking About?

The X-ray confirmed it: another victory for the skateboard. The seven-year-old in Minor Trauma had broken his distal radius.

"Well, it looks like Bobby is going to need a cast. He's fractured his wrist."

The boy's mother heaved a whistling sigh of relief. "Thank heaven. We were worried it was broken."

Broken, cracked, fractured—different terms for the same thing, but frequently confusing for a lot of us.

The same is true when we talk about *cholesterol.*

"Yeah, my doctor told me I have problems with my cholesterol and that I need to do something about it."

What exactly does that mean? Is her *total cholesterol* elevated? Or is her *HDL* low? Or is it a combination of things?

Technically, the proper term should be *lipids,* which includes cholesterol, HDL, LDL, VLDL, as well as triglycerides (more about each of these in a moment). And yes, we can have problems with each of these lipids—individually or collectively. Confusing? Sure it is. But we're going to walk through this, and by the time we're finished, you should have a good understanding of your lipids, why those numbers are important, and how you can take control of this important part of your overall health.

Let's start with the components of a basic lipid panel—the studies your physician routinely orders as part of your blood work. We'll look at these in more detail a little later, but for right now, it's important to understand the different parts of this panel.

Before we start, though, let's clear up a little confusion regarding the idea of "fasting blood work" versus "nonfasting." Most patients and a lot of physicians think that in order for your blood work to be accurate, you need to have fasted for some amount of time prior to having a sample drawn. Typically that period is eight to twelve hours. You can drink water or black coffee, but you can't have anything to eat or much to drink.

Important? Not really, unless you're worried about a person's glucose level. If that's the case, a *fasting* blood sugar is an important piece of information. But when it comes to measuring your lipids, fasting is not a critical factor. Your cholesterol, LDL, and HDL numbers are basically steady state—they don't fluctuate during the day, like your blood sugar does. So if you eat a double cheeseburger with fries an hour before having your blood drawn, it won't affect your total cholesterol. Over time it will, if you do that every day. That steady state will gradually creep up. But you can still get a valid measurement if you've had something to eat during the past eight to twelve hours.

The one lipid component that can change with food intake is your triglyceride level. When that double cheeseburger hits your stomach and small intestine, fat is rapidly absorbed and quickly enters your bloodstream, pushing that number up. It will come back down, but it can be misleading and not representative of your normal level.

So the bottom line: if you slip up and have some cereal or a bagel for breakfast, you can still have your lipids tested. If you've eaten a lot of fat (and who should be doing that?), the answer might be different, and you might have to return another day for your blood work.

Now, back to that lipid panel. What are all those numbers? First is your *cholesterol*. We're all familiar with this one. In fact, it may be the only one most of us pay any attention to. We'll be considering later how these measurements and calculations are actually made, but for right now, we just need to get a handle on the terminology. The cholesterol number is just that—the actual level of the cholesterol molecule in your bloodstream.

Now, here's where things get a little tricky. The next number reported is usually your *HDL*. You probably know this as your "good cholesterol," right? Well, not exactly. This is where we as healthcare providers have added to the potential for confusion. HDL is not really a type of cholesterol at all. It is **H**igh **D**ensity **L**ipoprotein. It is one of our lipids, to be sure, but it's a lipoprotein composed of some fat (*lipo*) and protein. The HDL molecule is small and tightly packed, hence the "high density" part of its name. The biochemistry here goes like this: cholesterol doesn't dissolve in our blood serum and needs a vehicle to transport it throughout our bodies. The HDL molecule is one of those vehicles. Cholesterol is bound to the HDL particle and is then able to be transported through the bloodstream and into various cells and tissues. This is true for all the lipoproteins, of which there are several. We refer to it as the "good cholesterol" for several reasons, which we'll look at later.

Next on the lab slip is the *LDL* value. And guess what? It's another lipoprotein. This time, the molecule is larger and more loosely put together, giving us the name **L**ow **D**ensity **L**ipoprotein. Again, it's not a type of cholesterol but another of those vehicles that carry cholesterol around. This is the "bad" one, and its reputation is well-earned.

Most labs report the *VLDL*—the **V**ery **L**ow **D**ensity **L**ipoprotein. You can use your imagination here, and you'll be right. It's even more loosely constructed than the LDL molecule and is also another cholesterol vehicle, usually present in much smaller amounts than your HDL or LDL.

And now we come to the *triglyceride* number. Triglycerides are important for a number of reasons, including the transfer of fats to and from adipose tissue (our fat cells and fatty tissue) to various destinations, such as the liver. The triglyceride molecule is composed of a basic unit called glycerol, which is then attached to three fatty acids. These fatty acids are relatively simple chains of carbon atoms, varying in length and in the way the carbon atoms are bonded together. This is where a little chemistry comes into play again, but bear with me—it's important.

Each carbon atom can form a certain number of bonds with a hydrogen molecule. When the carbon atoms of a chain of fatty acid have all their possible bonds occupied by a hydrogen molecule, it is said to be *saturated*. Sound familiar? And when some of these bonds remain empty, the fatty acid is *unsaturated*. If it's just one space, it's *monounsaturated*. And if a lot are empty, we have a *polyunsaturated* fat. It's as simple as that. Saturated fats and oils, and unsaturated fats and oils.

Examples of saturated fats are those found in cream, cheese, butter, coconut, cottonseed, and palm kernel oil. Generally, if it's animal fat, it's probably saturated fat. Unsaturated oils and fats can either be mono or polyunsaturated. The monounsaturated variety is found in whole milk products, olives, and avocados. These fats have been shown to reduce LDL levels and raise HDL levels in our bodies, and are an important part of the Mediterranean Diet. Polyunsaturated fats are found in nuts, seeds, fish, and leafy vegetables. These fats and oils have been thought to be the healthiest for us, but our knowledge in this area is expanding and current recommendations are changing. What *hasn't* changed is the evidence that we should significantly lower our ingestion of the saturated varieties.

What about *trans fats*? The evidence here is overwhelming. These are bad actors and known causes of heart disease, hypertension, and even type 2 diabetes. These are usually liquid oils that have been chemically altered so that they are completely hydrogenated—saturated. They don't occur naturally to any extent, but beginning around 1902, this hydrogenating process was found to alter various fats and oils, making them very attractive to the food industry. At room temperatures, fats could now remain solid (margarine, shortening), but then return to a soft or liquid state when heated or eaten.

Their use exploded, and a huge business was born. It took many decades for us to learn that this unnatural fatty complex was killing us. Fortunately, most countries have banned trans fats, and though the US lags behind in this regard, we are gradually seeing this deadly and totally unnecessary chemical disappear from our fast-food chains, restaurants, and grocery stores.

We've covered the basic glossary of our lipids. Later we'll take a look at each of these in a little more detail.

8

Now About Your Numbers…

Okay, so we know something about all those things listed on our lipid panel report. The next step is to understand what's high, what's low, and where those numbers *should* be. It's important to remember that from time to time these recommendations may change, based on emerging research or the results of some huge, overwhelmingly significant study. As of this printing, the numbers and recommendations given here have been pretty much the same for a while, and they are good guidelines and targets for us to consider.

But here's something else to remember—these numbers and levels are somewhat arbitrary. They are based on our best estimates and past experience. The reality is we just don't know the specific level above which everyone will develop problems or the magic number below which your arteries will remain pristine. We just do our best.

Before we begin, we need to consider how these numbers are determined and how they get to that printed piece of paper.

We are able to *directly* measure the level of cholesterol in our blood, as well as the amount of HDL. These are steady-state numbers and not affected by our last meal. Our triglycerides are also measured directly and should be measured while fasting. Most people define *fasting* as nothing to eat or drink for the previous ten to twelve hours, though water and black coffee are fine.

That leaves us with the LDL and VLDL numbers. These particles are *not* measured directly, but are calculated—determined by a couple of formulae. They *can* be measured directly if needed, but the cost is significant and usually unnecessary. Since the LDL is calculated and not measured, it can be skewed when the triglyceride value is high (usually more than 400 mg/dl) and most labs will simply not report a number when that's the case. But if your triglycerides are *that* high, you've got other things to be worried about.

Here's another little piece of information, one that can cause some confusion. Your lipid levels can vary based on several different and unexpected factors. The first is simply lab variation and the nature of testing in general. If you have the same sample of blood tested three different times, you will almost certainly get three different numbers. This is true for our lipids, as well as our blood sugar, hemoglobin, and almost anything else we want to measure. Usually this is a small, insignificant variance, but with your cholesterol, it can vary 5 to 10 mg/dl. That's why you shouldn't get too worked up (or pat yourself on the back) for a change in this range. We're looking for larger movements in those numbers.

And how about this—your *posture*, as well as stress and minor illness, can affect your numbers. And then there's the impact of the season of the year. Total cholesterol peaks in the winter and bottoms out in the summer. Fortunately, these changes are not significant—somewhere around 4 to 5 mg/dl—but they can be confusing and need to be kept in mind. And you thought this part was going to be straightforward.

Okay, now for our *total cholesterol* level. 200 mg/dl and below is considered normal, while a value between 200 and 239 is considered borderline high. Anything above that is abnormally high and a problem. Generally, the lower this number the better, though a value that's *too* low is associated with poor health and increased mortality. That threshold is thought to be around 75 mg/dl, and is usually caused by poor diet, malnutrition, starvation, or some significant disease process.

Now we move on to our *HDL*, the "good cholesterol." Again, this is measured directly, and should be at least 40 mg/dl. Numbers below that are associated with an increased risk for heart disease, while higher numbers—especially those above 60 or 70—are associated with markedly reduced risk.

Some labs report a cholesterol/HDL ratio—simply dividing the total cholesterol by the HDL. Most experts do not use this to manage their patients with lipid abnormalities, so it's not something we're going to be concerned with here. Just be aware that we might see it on our lab report, but know that the individual numbers are what we need to be addressing.

Next on the report is the *LDL* – the "bad boy," and the one that deservedly gets the most attention. Because it's so important and because we're learning more about its association with heart disease, the LDL target number has changed over the past few years. The maximum acceptable level is 130 mg/dl, but the *optimal* value is somewhere between 100 and 110. Most experts recommend a level of 100 if a person is at high risk for developing heart disease (family history, other vascular diseases, diabetes, hypertension) and 70 if there is a very high risk (the same risk factors but worse, and with a history of a known cardiovascular event). I want all of my patients to be below 100, and at or below 70 if at all possible.

The *VLDL* should be somewhere between 5 and 40 mg/dl, but this number is not extensively used at this time, since it varies with the amount of fat and triglycerides in our serum.

And that brings us to the *triglyceride* level—the amount of fats floating around in our blood. These numbers are being adjusted a little as well, but the general consensus is that a normal value is 150 mg/dl or less. Borderline high is 150 to 199, and high would be 200 to 499. Anything above that is very high and dangerous.

So there are your numbers. Get your total cholesterol, LDL, and triglycerides low, and your HDL high.

But how often do we need to check these, and when do we start? Again, no clear answer at this point, but most pediatricians are getting a baseline lipid panel on their kids before the age of ten. Certainly all of us need to know our numbers before the age of twenty, and beyond that, the frequency of testing depends on a couple of things. If our numbers are out of line, we will need annual testing—maybe even more frequently, especially if we're adjusting medications or lifestyles. Otherwise, if you're fortunate to have good numbers, testing your lipids every five years may well suffice.

The bottom line though is you gotta know your numbers.

What Diet Is Best for Me?

I wish there were an easy answer to this question. It would make things a lot simpler for my patients and for me. The reality, though, is there is no one single answer, no singular, supreme guideline that works for everyone. Each of us is different, with unique metabolisms, assorted health conditions, and maybe most importantly, distinctive tastes and preferences. Oh, and we each come with our own set of weaknesses, especially concerning what we put into our stomachs.

However, there *is* good news here. We continue to learn more about how our bodies handle the three major food groups—proteins, fats, and carbohydrates. And we continue to learn how what we eat can either improve our health or have a negative impact. We now know some acquired diseases are definitely connected to what and how much we eat.

Because of this ongoing research and expanding knowledge, we are able to make recommendations regarding specific diets and dietary trends. Later we'll look at some of these, but for now, there is significant agreement with the following:

- Limit total fat to 30 percent of your daily caloric intake.
- Avoid trans fats like the plague.
- Olive oil is preferable to most other cooking oils.
- Daily cholesterol intake should be less than 300 mgs.
- Avoid sugar-sweetened beverages.

- Avoid sugar like the plague.
- Daily water intake should be six to eight 8-ounce glasses.
- Limit naturally sweetened juice (no added sugar) to 4-6 ounces per day.
- Increase daily fiber intake to 25-40 grams each day.
- Limit salt intake.
- Limit or avoid processed foods.
- Limit carbohydrate intake as much as possible.
- Include lean meats and fish while reducing animal fat.

Most of these just make common sense, and while there are a lot of "limits" in that list, those are things we need to watch closely. We'll talk a little later about why these are important. But for right now, these are some general guidelines to keep in mind.

Or if you like your guidelines even simpler, you could heed this warning by Theresa M. Davis, a board-certified advance practice registered nurse: "If it comes out of a can or a box or a wrapper or through a fast-food window, it eventually is going to kill you."

How each of us decides to eat and what diet we choose to follow is a unique decision. But it's an important one, with far-reaching and significant implications. That's why we're going to spend some time considering this topic.

Why Low-Fat Diets Just Don't Work

There are a couple of cornerstones when it comes to managing elevated lipids, and our diet—what we put into our bodies—is arguably the most important. Sadly, it's also the most difficult to get our hands around. (Getting our hands around a double-cheeseburger is much easier.) But we haven't had a lot of guidance in this regard. In fact, somebody's got some 'splainin' to do.

In the early 1980s, the medical community was beginning to piece together the connection between elevated cholesterol levels and the risk of developing heart disease. The incidence of cardiovascular disease was rapidly rising, hand-in-hand with the obesity epidemic. Something needed to be done. Cholesterol—and by association red meats, bacon, fatty foods (especially saturated fats)—became the whipping boy of a progressive movement to improve the health of our nation and reduce the rampant heart disease that was taking its toll in lives lost and dollars spent.

But we were wrong. It turns out the real culprit here was not cholesterol and fatty foods, but carbohydrates, and more specifically, *high glycemic carbohydrates.*

Let's take a look at the evidence. When we began to eliminate cholesterol (and fat) from our diets, we had to replace it with something. That something became carbohydrates—grains, cereal, pasta, bread, potatoes. After all, we have only three categories of nutrients to choose from: fats, carbs, and proteins. We have largely chosen carbs—the comfort foods—and we've become addicted. Cholesterol became the persona non grata and "cholesterol free" became, and still is, the mantra of the food industry.

But let's get back to the evidence, and it's pretty sobering. We've been pushing this "fat free" business for almost forty years. Surely by now we would be seeing some positive results. What about the incidence of heart disease? Has it plummeted? Of course not. We may be seeing a bit of a leveling off, but this is thought to be due to a multitude of factors, including better treatments, more awareness and screening, and a gradual reduction in the rate of cigarette smoking. But we're certainly not seeing the precipitous drop that had been hoped for.

What about the obesity epidemic? After all, obesity is closely tied to the onset of premature heart disease, as well as to the development of several other major problems. We all know the answer to this question—the epidemic continues to explode, and not just in this country. Over the past thirty years, the worldwide incidence of obesity has increased by almost 30 percent in adults. Alarmingly, that number rises to almost 50 percent in our children. One out of every two. But where is this happening? We know we have a problem in the US, but in what other parts of the world are we seeing this explosion of obesity?

The World Health Organization (WHO) has recently published data that list the ten countries that account for more than half of the earth's obese population. In addition to the United States, those nations are India, China, Brazil, Russia, Indonesia, Mexico, Egypt, Germany, and Pakistan. Some of these might surprise you, but that's what WHO has reported.

Many factors are involved in this epidemic, including a progressive decrease in the amount of regular physical exercise we are getting, and in this country at least, the pervasiveness of fast-food restaurants. We're just not eating right. But it's not the red meat that's doing this; it's the relentless move to reduce fats in our diet, which we've replaced with more high glycemic-index carbs. What are we talking about here?

Let's start with the *glycemic index*. This is a system of comparing the relative amounts of sugar in various foods and how rapidly they release glucose into our bloodstreams. The higher the index rating, the faster glucose is released, the more rapid the rise of our blood sugar levels, and the more insulin required to get that level under control. A lower index rating still releases glucose into our system, but at a more controlled, manageable rate.

For the sake of simplicity, this index uses pure glucose as the gold standard and assigns it a value of 100. Everything else is pegged to this number. Here are some examples:

- Low glycemic-index (GI) foods—55 or less

  Avocados, beans, almonds, peanuts, whole intact grains

- Medium GI foods—56-69

  Grape juice, raisins, honey, not intact whole grains, bananas

- High GI foods—70-100

  Whole wheat bread, corn flakes (92!), pretzels, bagels, potatoes

If you take a close look here, you won't see any meats or fats listed. Remember, proteins and fats don't contain any carbs, and fruits and vegetables don't contain any cholesterol. The GI of corn flakes is surprising, as is that for a baked potato (85). Table sugar comes in at 58, placing it in the medium range.

Why is this important? In a nutshell (no cholesterol here), high glycemic foods trigger a rapid release of insulin, which does a lot of bad things. It tells the body to make and store fat for that potential rainy day, which we all know is not coming. In those of us who get little exercise, this body fat is deposited around our trunk—a pattern that we now know is associated with hyperlipidemia and an increased risk of heart disease. Additionally, high GI foods, because of rapidly rising and falling blood-sugar levels, trigger a hunger response, causing us to eat more (usually more carbs) and gain more weight.

If all of this is valid, we would be seeing an increase in obesity in this country. And guess what?

If you want to gain a deeper understanding of this problem, I recommend two books. The first is *Grain Brain,* written by David Perlmutter, a neurologist (Little, Brown and Company, 2013). The other is *Wheat Belly* by William Davis, a cardiologist (Rodale Books, 2011). Be prepared—they're not for the faint of heart.

So if our current low-fat/high-carb approach is killing us, what are we supposed to be eating? And how do we make that change?

It might not be as difficult as you think.

The Low-Carb Approach

While it's true that we all put our pants on one leg at a time, those pants are different sizes, shapes, and colors. We are a little different, and one size doesn't fit all.

The same is true when it comes to determining the best diet. We're all a little different, and one diet doesn't fit all. There *is* something that comes close to being a constant though, and that is that we all (some more than others) need to limit our carbohydrate intake.

But what's so bad about carbs? Why the rap against our "comfort foods"? Let's start with the real culprit here—*insulin*. This is something we really need to understand.

As we mentioned earlier, our body needs energy to grow and survive. We get that from three sources: carbohydrates, proteins, and fats. We are able to derive energy from each of these classes of nutrients, but carbs are the easiest, quickest source—and in the long run, the most harmful. That's because in order to utilize the energy in carbs, we must have the action of the hormone insulin.

Insulin is made in the "beta cells" of the pancreas, and is a relatively simple chain of fifty-one amino acids. Its release is signaled by the presence of carbohydrates in our bloodstream. When this process is initiated, insulin circulates throughout the body, seeking and attaching itself to insulin receptors. These are chemical binders located on the membranes of "target cells," and once the insulin molecule combines with this receptor, the hormone is able to exert its actions, which are many.

Insulin directly or indirectly affects almost every tissue in our body. These actions are complex and interwoven, but right now, we're going to mainly consider how it interacts with glucose and how it affects the production of energy. It does this by its action on three tissues: the liver, muscles, and adipose tissue (fat).

Glucose—the simplest and most basic sugar—can be immediately used for energy throughout the body, or it can be stored in the liver as glycogen. Once stored, this complex of modified glucose molecules can be readily and rapidly used as an energy source when needed. Lastly, excess glucose can be converted into fat and stored in our adipose tissue. Getting the energy out of this fat is a more complex process than burning available glucose and it takes a little longer. That's why our bodies first burn and deplete the available glucose and then our glycogen stores before finally turning to our adipose tissue. And that's one of the reasons it's so hard to get rid of unwanted fat.

Now let's consider how insulin impacts our metabolism of glucose. Remember the glycemic index? Every carbohydrate we put into our body eventually becomes glucose—some quicker than others. But even the highly touted complex carbohydrates end up as circulating glucose. All carbs, from simple to complex, end up as glucose and all activate the release of insulin.

The first thing this hormone does is move glucose into the cells of various tissues. As we noted earlier, this is done by attaching itself to the cell's insulin receptor. You may have heard of or even been told that you have some degree of "insulin resistance." A cell's insulin receptor is the location where that resistance takes place. The receptors seem to wear down over time after repeatedly being called into action due to a persistently high-carb diet. More and more insulin is required to activate the signal and allow glucose to enter the cell.

You see where this leads—more and more insulin required to do the same amount of work and handle the same sugar load. The beta cells of the pancreas finally say, "I'm getting too old for this," and stop working. And that condition? Right—adult-onset diabetes. If this theory is correct, we should have an epidemic of diabetes on our hands given our colossal consumption of carbohydrates. And guess what. We do.

But back to the actions of insulin. It drives glucose into the cells of the liver, where it stimulates the formation of glycogen. It drives glucose into muscle cells, where it can be immediately burned for energy. And it drives glucose into the cells of our adipose tissue, where it promotes the storage of triglycerides in our fat cells.

This is a good time to consider why insulin has been called "the hormone of plenty." When we have plenty to eat, and a lot of glucose circulating throughout our bodies, insulin rapidly converts some of this to needed energy. The rest is stored away for a rainy day in the form of glycogen or as fat. (As most of us can attest, we have a significant capacity for storing fat, usually in places we would rather not.)

The problem with this rainy day business is that, in this country, that day never comes. Three not-so-square meals a day is the norm, with a few snacks thrown in for good measure. But our pancreas doesn't know that, and each time we load ourselves with carbs, insulin does what it's supposed to do: burn sugar and store fat—taking advantage of this moment of plenty and preparing for more austere, less plentiful times.

Along the way, it can elevate our blood pressures, damage the walls of our arteries, and interfere with the normal clotting that takes place in these vessels, leading to the formation of atherosclerotic plaques. There is even emerging evidence that excess levels of insulin may be associated with the development of several cancers, including those of the colon, ovary, and breast.

Lest I give you a completely one-sided view of this essential hormone, insulin does some important and beneficial things. It does handle glucose for us, and it is important in the growth process and the formation of proteins. The problem is that it was never intended to handle the kinds of carbohydrate loads we throw at our pancreas.

The bottom line: we all need to reduce the amount of carbohydrates we consume. It doesn't matter whether we're talking about whole grains, complex carbs, or multigrain whatever. We need to know the carb content of what we're putting into our bodies and lower it.

That brings up a frequent and important question: What constitutes a low-carb diet? How many daily grams of carbs is okay?

Some general but useful guidelines are available here. Robert Atkins (of the Atkins Diet fame) would tell us that the cutoff should be 30 to 45 grams per day. That's hard, considering that one piece of whole-wheat bread has 23 grams, and one medium banana contains 26 grams.

A more realistic approach would be to target 60 or so grams per day, knowing that it's impossible to identify and eliminate every single carb from your diet. And we don't want to, anyway. A certain amount of carbs is essential for our well-being. We just need to find a way to limit their intake and restore the balanced diet our systems were designed to handle. It won't take something as drastic as the Atkins Diet, though that might be a good place to start for a couple of weeks. Fortunately, we have some effective alternatives, diets that will get the job done and that we can live with long-term.

We'll take a look at some of these next.

(For a great discussion of our hunter-gatherer origins, I recommend the book *Protein Power* by Michael R. Eades and Mary Dan Eades. And for a complete discussion of the importance of low-carb diets, there are two books you should look at: *60 Ways to Lower Your Blood Sugar* by Dennis Pollock and *The New Sugar Busters!* by H. Leighton Steward and others. These are all great resources and will help clarify the mistakes and myths of the past few decades regarding what we should and should not be eating.)

12

Low Carb:
A Case in Point

"Well, Richard, that sounds more like the Mayo Fatso Diet to me."

Richard, my medical partner of more than thirty years, had just told me about a diet he had been on for the previous six months. This was fourteen years ago, and the Mayo Clinic Diet was making the Internet rounds. It was a one-page flyer with a list of acceptable foods and another of those strictly forbidden. A sample diet was included, with instructions for what you should eat for each meal, including breakfast. It had all the trappings of the low-carbohydrate Atkin's Diet, with a few modifications. I was skeptical.

"Let me get this straight. Eggs and bacon every morning, with cheese if you want. And as much as you want."

"That's right," he said. "Just no bread, no potatoes, and no grits."

"And you lost weight?"

"I've been on the diet for six months and I've lost ten pounds."

That wasn't much, but Richard didn't need to lose a lot of weight.

"The most important thing about this diet is what it did for my lipid levels. My total cholesterol was around 220, and now it's 175. And my LDL dropped from 115 to less than 80."

"That's impressive." I studied the info sheet and wondered where bacon fit into all of this.

"But the best thing is what happened to my HDL. I couldn't get it above 40, no matter what I did. I exercised, took a bunch of supplements, but it wouldn't budge. And I didn't want to start taking prescription meds unless I absolutely had to. But after a month, my HDL was 82, and it hasn't gone down since."

"Your HDL is 82? That's amazing." It *was* amazing, and one of the highest levels I had ever encountered.

My own numbers flashed through my brain. Total cholesterol 210. LDL around 100. HDL 40. I had tried the same things Richard described—running five miles a day, working out on top of that, and taking flush-free niacin (which still left me red-faced). Nothing worked. My HDL wouldn't budge, and I convinced myself it must be a genetic problem.

"On top of all that, Robert, my blood pressure came down about ten points. Might be the weight loss, but I think it has something to do with this diet. You really restrict your carbohydrate intake and eat as much of most vegetables and protein as you want."

"And the bacon?"

Richard chuckled. "I stopped most of that after a week or so and stuck with lean meats—chicken, fish, lean beef. That part's easy. Actually, the whole thing is pretty easy. And it works. You need to give it a try, at least for a month. Check your labs first, and then in four weeks. If your lipids aren't better, you can call me and tell me I'm crazy. But that won't happen."

"Hmm…" I stared at the piece of paper and shook my head.

"What have you got to lose? Four weeks, that's all it will take. You're gonna thank me."

"We'll see."

It took a couple of weeks before I decided to give this diet a try. Several of our staff members had started it and were consistently losing weight. While I would be happy with losing a few pounds, I was more interested in my lipid levels. And with my blood pressure. It had slowly crept upwards, hovering around 130/90. Not terrible, but it needed to be lower.

All right. Why not give it a try?

I decided if I was going to do this thing, I would follow it to the letter. Every morning it was two fried eggs with cheese and bacon strips. After a while, I eliminated the bacon and replaced it with turkey and lean ham. Much less guilt.

And I picked up a book titled *Protein Power* by Michael Eades and Mary Dan Eades, a husband and wife team. They explained the theory behind the low-carb/high-protein diet, and it made sense. I soon found myself questioning my dietary habits and dogma. High cholesterol? Cut fat out of your diet. Stop eating beef and eggs and cheese. Replace those evil things with whole-wheat pasta, whole-grain breads, and baked potatoes. The problem with that approach—it just doesn't work. Eades and Eades explained why that was so, and laid it out in a convincing fashion. And while I ate my eggs and cheese, I started thinking.

It seemed the magic number for a low-carb diet was somewhere around 60 grams of carbs a day. That's not much. It's a target, and the reality will be somewhere higher than that. We need carbs to live and function properly, and we'll get them in unexpected places. Again, 60 grams is a target.

Let's see—what had my standard breakfast been before this? Following my old dogma, I had tried to eliminate as much fat and cholesterol as possible. A large glass of orange juice, one plain bagel, and a bowl of cereal with 1 percent skim milk. A little cholesterol in the milk, but not much. And then a heaping tablespoon of wheat germ, just because. A quick tally of the carbs in these foods and...

Good grief! I had blown close to three days of my carb target in one sitting. This breakfast contained very little cholesterol but almost 150 grams of carbohydrates! If Eades and Eades (and my partner) were correct, it was obvious why my lipids never improved. And why I couldn't lose those elusive ten pounds. Or why my blood pressure flirted just beyond the normal range.

Four weeks later, I had my answer. No, I had my *answers.*

Just as Richard had done, I lost those ten pounds. And my blood pressure dropped to 120/78. I had my blood drawn and waited. A few days later, our lab tech brought me the results, shaking her head as she walked into my office.

"What's the matter?" I got up and walked around the desk.

"You're not going to believe this." She had my chart in her hands and was comparing these new numbers with those of a month earlier. "Take a look."

My total cholesterol was now 175, and my LDL, the bad cholesterol, was down to 84. A great number. I stared at my HDL, not believing what screamed at me from the piece of paper—83. Incredible. No amount of exercise had budged this number in over ten years.

"Dr. Lesslie, those are great numbers," she said. "I need to get my husband in here and let you get him started on this diet."

Since that day, I've recommended the low-carb/high-protein diet to many of my patients. Most of them have been successful with it, and a few, for various reasons, have found it too difficult to maintain. It's not for everyone, but the concepts are solid and founded in fact and experience and a growing mountain of evidence.

The Mayo Fatso Diet turned out to work after all. Oh, and please pass me the bacon.

13

A Couple of Diet Options

As you can see by now, a lot of questions surround the issue of what we need to be eating. In our clinic, we are frequently asked about our recommendations to help with weight loss and, to a lesser extent, to help manage lipid disorders and blood-sugar problems. Again, one size doesn't fit all, and if there is a magic wand somewhere, I've yet to find it.

From a previous chapter, we've considered the failure of a low-fat diet as a cure-all. That leaves us with a couple of viable choices, and we'll discuss those here.

First is the Mediterranean Diet. It should be understood that there is no single definition for this diet, and in fact, the word *Mediterranean* might be somewhat of a misnomer. The name is used to refer to a way of eating that is high in fruits, vegetables, whole grains, beans, nuts (especially walnuts), and seeds. Additionally, there is low to moderate intake of fish and poultry and little red meat. Wine consumption (low to moderate amounts) is acceptable, and olive oil is a mainstay. There are numerous books on the subject, as well as dietary plans and menus. But does it make sense?

Several large and recent studies indicate the answer is yes. When compared to a low-fat diet, the Mediterranean Diet significantly reduces the rates of cardiovascular events (strokes, heart attacks, and cardiovascular deaths). Interestingly, it also appears to reduce the development of Parkinson's and Alzheimer's diseases. And this diet also appears to lower the chances of developing type 2 diabetes.

Since the inclusion of olive oil is foundational to this diet, let's take a moment to clear up some confusion. If you're Italian or a Californian, this is probably old hat and you can skip this section. But for the rest of us, we find the labeling of olive oil to be perplexing. Let's take a stab at it.

On the grocery store shelf, we're faced with multiple olive oil products of various descriptions and costs. We'll start with the lowest quality—"pure olive oil." This is almost always *refined*, meaning that some chemical process (maybe only the use of charcoal) has been employed to remove impurities that adversely affect the flavor. This is the cheapest olive oil on the shelf.

Next is "virgin olive oil." It can't contain any refined oil and may have a free fatty-acid content up to 1.5 or 2 percent. This amount of acidity affects the flavor of the oil, making it good but not great.

The great stuff would be "extra virgin olive oil." Again, no refined oil here, and the free fatty-acid content can't exceed .8 percent. This is the highest quality and best tasting olive oil. It's probably the best for you as well.

What about "cold pressed" or "cold extracted" on the label? This has to do with how hot the oil is allowed to get during processing. To be called "cold pressed," the temperature can't exceed 80 degrees F. This supposedly preserves the natural nutrients and flavors.

There, now you're an expert and can impress your friends at your next dinner party. What seems clear is that we all need to consume more olive oil in our diets and use it to replace other cooking oils.

Another diet, the South Beach Diet, was developed by a cardiologist and dietician as an alternative to the low-fat diet, which just wasn't working. This diet has become very popular, and you can find a lot of books and plans on its use. What sets it apart from other diets is the focus on "good carbs" versus "bad carbs."

The good carbs are those with a lower glycemic index: most vegetables, beans, and whole grains. And the bad carbs are on the other end of the glycemic index spectrum: processed grains, sugars, potatoes.

As you can see, this diet is not really focused on being low carb, and I'm not sure the body can differentiate very well between a good carb and a bad one. Mounting medical evidence agrees. Yet the South Beach Diet does move us away from the exclusion of meat and fat. That's a good thing, since we know that strategy just doesn't work.

Last, we need to address the DASH Diet. I'm asked about this from time to time in our office, and I tell my patients that this is not really a weight-loss diet or a means of lowering your cholesterol. The acronym stands for **D**ietary **A**pproach to **S**top **H**ypertension, and it's effective in doing that. It stresses the inclusion of fruits and vegetables, while limiting the amount of low-fat dairy products and lean meats. It's also rich in potassium, magnesium, and calcium—minerals that are efficient in lowering blood pressure. And as we noted, strict adherence to this diet is an effective weapon in the battle to control blood pressure.

Where does that leave us? Is there one specific diet we should try? Probably not. The advice I give to my patients is to familiarize themselves with the key elements of the Mediterranean Diet and make some minor alterations to it. This includes more lean meats and less grains. Nuts are great for snacking, especially walnuts and almonds. And as already mentioned, olive oil (the extra virgin variety if you can afford it) should occupy a preeminent place in our pantry.

Before we move on from the importance of what we eat for controlling our lipids, one important point needs to be made. If your cholesterol/LDL/triglycerides are elevated and your healthcare provider advises you to stick to a low-fat/low-cholesterol diet, it's time to find a new provider. That kind of diet won't work, and may very well make matters worse. Remind him or her that several large studies comparing low-fat to low-carb diets clearly give the thumbs-up to low carbohydrates. Fewer deaths, less heart disease, less diabetes, and more and sustainable weight loss. They should know better.

14

Give Me the Details, Doc

Your Total Cholesterol

Admit it. The word *cholesterol* doesn't evoke a lot of pleasant thoughts. Probably just the opposite. We attach many negative feelings and emotions to this innocent molecule, through no fault of our own. We've been taught to do that. Yet, without cholesterol, life as we know it would not exist.

That's right—cholesterol is essential for all animal life and a very important building block in many critical internal processes. The most important of these has to do with serving as a structural component in cell membranes—the things that hold us together. In addition to that, cholesterol is a vital component of such things as bile acids (essential for digestion), steroid hormones (such as cortisol, estrogens, testosterone, and others), as well as important vitamins (D, A, E, and K). In other words, we can't live without it. It's only when its level becomes too high in our bloodstreams, or the various components that transport it are out of whack, that we have a problem.

But where does it come from? Double cheeseburgers and bacon, right? Wrong. Contrary to what most of us think, dietary intake of cholesterol has little to do with the amount of cholesterol in our bloodstream and body.

As an aside, my editor shared with me that in the early '90s he participated in a diet study led by Dr. William Connor, coauthor of *The New*

American Diet (1986) and a researcher at Oregon Health and Science University. The study consisted of a controlled diet in three phases where the fat in the foods the study participants were given to eat remained constant but the cholesterol in the food was low one month, high the next, and moderate for the third. My editor's blood cholesterol was tested weekly, and there was no obvious correlation between dietary cholesterol and the cholesterol in his blood.

Most of what we ingest is chemically modified in our upper GI tract and poorly absorbed. So the majority of the cholesterol each of us carries around is manufactured throughout our bodies. Depending on a person's size, the amount varies between 35 and 100 grams (roughly between 1 and 3 ounces)—not much for something that demands so much of our attention.

This manufacturing process happens in most of our cells, forming those cell walls we talked about. But it especially occurs in the liver (around 25 percent overall), as well as in our adrenal glands and intestines. That's important to remember—the cholesterol we ingest when we eat animal products doesn't necessarily impact our blood levels. That is largely determined by other facets of our diets, as well as by our individual genetic makeups. Some of us just make more cholesterol than others. Doesn't seem fair, but that's the way it is. And that's one of the things that makes treating elevated lipid levels such a challenge—one size doesn't fit everyone. What works well for one person doesn't necessarily work at all for another. More about that later.

Here's another interesting fact about cholesterol, and one that should make us marvel at God's handiwork when he designed our complex and intricate bodies. The process of forming the cholesterol molecule (a relatively small and simple one, compared to other organic compounds) requires thirty-seven separate, distinct steps. *Thirty-seven!* And that's just for one of a multitude of the molecular building blocks that comprise our bodies and support our lives.

In addition to being fascinating, this fact is also very important. One of the very early steps in this process involves an enzyme (HMG-CoA reductase) to move the reaction forward. It's at this point that the statin drugs have their effect. They block this enzyme and stop the formation of cholesterol. You don't have to remember the name of the enzyme, but we'll be talking later about statins and how they work.

Once cholesterol is formed, it provides those vital functions we talked about earlier and is extensively recycled. This mainly happens in the liver, where the molecule is excreted back into the GI tract. Since it's not chemically altered as is the cholesterol in our food, more than half of it is absorbed through the small intestine and back into our bloodstreams. This is another important fact when it comes to trying to lower our lipid levels. If we can reduce the amount that is reabsorbed, we should be able to reduce the levels in our blood, and that's exactly what happens. We'll be looking at that when we consider specific treatment options.

Let's get back to the dietary sources of cholesterol and fats, and how that impacts the regulation of cholesterol levels in our blood.

The typical American diet is way too high in animal fats—complex mixtures of triglycerides and smaller amounts of cholesterol. Because of that, all foods containing animal fat will contain varying amounts of cholesterol. We know most of the major sources: beef, pork, cheese, egg yolks, some types of fish, and shrimp. But remember, it's not the amount of cholesterol you ingest that drives up your cholesterol level. That number is determined by multiple factors, including the amount of other fats you ingest, as well as the amount of carbohydrates in your diet.

The exact mechanism of this regulation is not completely understood, but we do know that when our levels of cholesterol go up, the cells of our bodies stop manufacturing it. And when the levels drop, the opposite occurs. We also know that we can overwhelm these regulatory mechanisms by dietary indiscretion—a polite term for eating too much bad stuff. Too much fat in our diets will change the amount of cholesterol our bodies manufacture, as well as the types of lipoproteins that carry it in our blood.

Now here's something that really aggravates me. How often do you pick up a bag of peanuts or some other plant or fruit product and read in bold print "Cholesterol-free!" Of course peanuts are cholesterol free, as are carrots and cucumbers and tomatoes and every other vegetable and fruit on this planet. It's only animal products that contain this molecule.

It is of interest, though, that some plants—peanuts and flax seeds for example—contain something called phytosterols. These are compounds that resemble cholesterol and are believed to compete with the cholesterol that is absorbed in our intestines. Hence these phytosterols and the foods that contain them are generally regarded as being healthy and useful in reducing some of the bad lipids in our bloodstreams. Several phytosterol supplements are available on the market, though there is no conclusive evidence that any of these are beneficial.

So there's the basic information about cholesterol. It's essential to our well-being while at the same time, when present in excess and in unhealthy forms, can lead to real and life-threatening problems. It requires a balance—one that we need to understand and manage.

15

Please Pass the Cardboard: The Importance of Fiber

As we grow older, it seems few things strike as much terror in our hearts as the fear of irregularity. It occupies many of our caregiver-patient conversations, is high on the list of concerns we have for our aging loved ones, and may even permeate our dreams (or nightmares, depending on your own experiences).

Unfortunately, the frequently rendered admonition to "increase your water and fiber intake" apparently isn't exciting enough, since few of us follow that sage advice.

Our daily intake of fiber is essential when it comes to the health of our GI tracts, especially our colons. And we now know that our dietary fiber intake is directly related to several significant health issues—especially our lipid levels and our individual risk for the development of colon cancer. While the prevention of cancer is important, elevated lipid levels and its associated increased incidence of heart disease is what we'll be considering here.

Let's start with a couple of simple definitions. When we speak of dietary fiber, we're referring to two types: soluble and insoluble. This ends up being important when we consider the effects that total fiber intake has on our health.

Soluble fiber is able to dissolve in water and in our GI tracts. There it forms a kind of gel that can partially ferment. Not a very pleasant thought, and if your family and friends consume a lot of foods that contain this type of fiber (pinto beans, for example), your personal experience might not be very pleasant either. But these gels do serve a purpose. They shield carbohydrates from the digestive process, thus preventing their absorption and breakdown into simple sugars and the problems involved with that.

Sources of soluble fiber include peas, soybeans, oats, rye, barley, broccoli, carrots, and onions. Nuts are also a good source of this type of fiber, with almonds topping the list.

Insoluble fiber doesn't dissolve in water and acts as a bulking agent in our GI tracts. This increased bulk not only helps with regularity, but it also gives us a sense of fullness, resulting in a reduced intake of food—both good things.

Sources of this type of fiber include whole-grain foods (*refined* grains have had the outer coat of bran removed and should be avoided), wheat and corn bran, nuts and seeds, potato skins as well as the skins of grapes, kiwis, and tomatoes. And yes, cardboard would be a good source as well.

As you can see, there is considerable overlap with these foods and their types of fiber. Most of what we eat contains a combination, thus making it necessary to simply list "dietary fiber" when labelling our foods.

Another thing you've probably noticed is that these are all plant sources. No beef or chicken or fish here. Our dietary fiber comes almost exclusively from vegetables and fruits. Let's take a look at some of those sources.

Most fruits (½ cup)—1.1 grams of fiber
Dark green vegetables (½ cup)—6.4 grams
Orange vegetables (½ cup)—2.4 grams
Cooked pinto beans (½ cup)—8.0 grams
Starchy vegetables (½ cup)—1.7 grams
Whole grains (1 ounce)—2.4 grams
Meat (1 ounce)—.1 gram

This gives us an idea of where to find our fiber. But how much is enough? The magic number keeps going higher, but at this point, the recommended daily amount is at least 30 grams/day. The goal drops a little as we get older (over the age of 50), but 30 is a good target, and you won't go wrong if you exceed it.

And the benefits of increased fiber in our diets? They are substantial. For instance, we know that individuals with diabetes have a much easier time managing their blood sugars if they increase their fiber intake. This has to do with that soluble/gel business, and the hiding of those carbohydrates in your GI tract. It works, and it's important.

The connection between dietary fiber intake and our lipid levels is also substantial. Some experts have quantified this connection, proposing that for each gram of fiber ingested, our LDL level may be reduced by a little more than 2 mgs. If you do the math, a significant increase in our fiber would be more effective than taking medication. But just how does that work?

Several factors are at play here, the most important being the "recycling" of lipids, especially cholesterol. The liver removes cholesterol and other lipids from our bloodstream and excretes them in the form of bile acids, which enter our gut and are reabsorbed. The presence of adequate amounts of fiber in our GI tract hinders this reabsorption and reduces the lipid levels in our blood. Some expensive medications are based entirely on this recycling disruption, but they don't work any better than the natural fiber God created.

"But can't I just take a pill? I don't like beans and spinach."

Sure, there are a bunch of fiber products on the market, a lot of which contain psyllium seed husks, an effective bulk enhancer. The downside is you don't get the benefits of the nutrients we find in fruits and vegetables. But yes, if you need to increase your fiber intake by incorporating a supplement into your diet, that works. The main thing is to work to achieve those recommended daily amounts we mentioned.

One thing that helps, as with *any* issue regarding our diets, is to keep a food journal. Sounds simple, but it requires a key element that is often in short supply—honesty. You have to make a note of everything you put in your mouth. No exceptions. This exercise can be very enlightening (or troubling, depending on your personal level of honesty). Such a journal will quickly point out problem areas in our diets as well as opportunities. If you just can't seem to lose weight, or your lipid or blood-sugar levels won't budge, keep a journal for a couple of weeks and share it with your healthcare provider. I always appreciate the effort my patients make with this, and welcome that level of involvement. We always find something to work on.

And when it comes to working on your fiber, keep in mind those daily goals and the readily available foods to help reach them. After all, wouldn't we rather be talking about our children and grandchildren than our colons?

16

Where's the Beef?

I grew up eating beef—sirloin on the grill, T-bones on rare and special occasions, roast beef after church on Sundays. And during medical school, we learned that if you pound rump steak, flank, and brisket long and hard enough, they might become sufficiently tender to eat. Later, there were the nuances of various marinades and creative ways of grilling.

So I'm no vegetarian. However, as I examine my eating habits over the past few years, I realize I am eating much less beef and a lot more chicken and fish. I'm not sure it's been a conscious decision—more likely a gradual evolution in preferences. Yet, the constant drumming to reduce fat and cholesterol in our diets has surely had an effect.

Since proteins are an essential part of our diets, and red meat (mainly beef and pork) is a significant source of this, what do we really know here—the good and the bad?

First, as we just stated, beef is an excellent source of protein. It's also a great source of iron, in a form that is quickly and easily digested and absorbed into our systems. And it contains significant amounts of vitamin B_{12} and zinc, both important nutrients, essential for our health. Red meat contains no carbohydrates and unfortunately adds very little dietary fiber.

But we know that beef also contains significant amounts of fat and cholesterol, depending on how lean the cut. Conventional wisdom has taught us that this will lead to elevated lipid levels and heart disease. Maybe not. We are learning that our lipid levels are affected by a lot of factors, not the least of which is our carbohydrate intake, and not necessarily by the fact that we consume red meat.

Here's the quandary: As with most things in life, it's all about moderation and balance. We can always overdo a good thing, and our human natures seem to be very adept at doing just that.

As an example of that balance, a recent large study looked at the consumption of beef and its effects on blood pressure and the health of blood vessels. The authors determined that the daily consumption of moderate amounts of beef actually helped reduce blood pressure levels and had no damaging effects on the lining of blood vessels. The operative word here is *moderate*, which the authors defined as a four-ounce serving (about the size of a deck of cards), probably not enough to satisfy most steakhouse patrons—or even hungry teenagers and adults at home. Still, daily consumption of this amount of beef was helpful in this particular study.

What else do we know about this moderation business? A previous study indicated that people who consume eight or more servings of beef a month (with a serving defined as six to seven ounces), when compared to individuals who had four servings a month, had a fivefold increase in the number of cardiac events over several years of study. That's a huge number, and something that should concern all of us.

Moderation it seems *is* the key. At present, that would be four, maybe five servings of beef a month, and those servings need to be five to six ounces only. That's going to take some getting used to for most of us. And don't forget about the lean part. Sometimes there's some confusion about this term, but the general guideline is that a three-ounce lean cut of meat should contain less than ten grams of total fat. A good rule of thumb is that most cuts of meat with "loin" in the name are probably lean—sirloin tip, top sirloin, pork tenderloin, and lamb loin chops.

The quandary doesn't end here, though. In spite of the positives of moderate beef consumption, there are some troubling negatives.

Growing evidence supports the connection between red and processed meats with an increased risk of developing colon, esophageal, liver, and prostate cancers. The data supporting this are substantial and impossible to overlook.

That's troubling. But more troubling may be the results of a large study recently published in the *British Medical Journal*. The authors tied the consumption of red and processed meat to the incidence of breast cancer. This is the second leading cancer in the US and the number one cancer for women, so we need to pay attention. The authors reported a significant increase in the risk of breast cancer for women who consumed a little more than one serving per day of red meat. As the number of servings went up, so did the risk. As further proof of the connection, the authors noted that women who consumed little red meat but more chicken and fish had a substantially smaller risk of developing this disease. That's the silver lining here—this increased risk of having breast cancer can easily be modified, just by changing one's diet.

So, where's the beef? Just where does red meat fit into a smart, healthy diet?

Unless the tide of medical research drastically turns (possible, but unlikely), we should rely less on red meat for our protein and more on chicken, fish, beans, and nuts. For the present, that would mean four moderate servings of lean red meat a month—no more than once a week.

Moderation—and balance.

17

The Dreaded Syndrome X: The Metabolic Syndrome

One in three. Take a look around you. According to some experts, one in three of us has or will develop this problem. That's a lot, and "Syndrome X" sounds pretty serious, so what are we talking about?

The term *metabolic syndrome* may be a little more appropriate and certainly a lot gentler. This actually *is* a metabolic issue, one that was first described seventy or eighty years ago and whose definition continues to be refined.

One thing for certain—this is real, and it has significant consequences. Those of us who bear this diagnosis have a significantly increased risk of developing cardiovascular disease (heart disease, strokes, and especially heart failure) and diabetes. Serious business, so how do I know if I have it?

Here's a list of five all-too-common medical conditions (all definitions are from the American Heart Association guidelines). If I have three of the five, I have the syndrome.

1. Abdominal (central) obesity—a waist circumference greater than 40 inches in men and 35 inches in women. Some experts describe this as "apple-shaped obesity," with adipose tissue accumulating mainly around the waist and trunk. We're not really sure why this is significant, but a clear connection exists between this type of obesity and the development of heart disease and diabetes.

2. Elevated blood pressure—blood pressure equal to or greater than

130/85 or use of medication for hypertension. The medication aspect here is interesting. Whenever I conduct a Department of Transportation certification for truck drivers, I routinely ask if there is any history of high blood pressure. The driver may have noted on his medical history form that he takes BP medications, but I need to ask anyway.

Often the driver will respond, "No, I don't have high blood pressure. I take medicine for that."

Excuse me? Of course he has hypertension. His normal reading on blood pressure meds doesn't erase that fact. The same thing holds true for a diabetic on medication. He or she still has diabetes. That's the reason for the "use of medication" in these definitions.

3. *Elevated fasting glucose*—equal to or greater than 100mg/dl or use of medication for diabetes. Here again, an elevated blood sugar or treatment for diabetes satisfies this definition.

4. *Elevated triglycerides*—equal to or greater than 150mg/dl.

5. *Reduced HDL* (the good cholesterol)—less than 40 mg/dl in men and 50 in women.

Three out of five of these is all it takes to qualify for the metabolic syndrome, and one in three Americans has it. These conditions are all very common and negatively impact our healthcare and enjoyment of living.

The causes of this disorder seem intuitively obvious. Some are just that, but others are more perplexing. While the exact mechanisms of this complex condition are not fully known, several interconnecting pathways shed light on its causes. Let's take a look.

Obesity (especially central obesity). This is a key feature of the syndrome, and a body mass index (BMI) of greater than 30 should alert a person and their caregiver to this problem. (For a brief definition of BMI and a handy calculator to determine your BMI, go to www.nhlbi.nih.gov/health/edu cational/lose_wt/BMI/bmicalc.htm.)

Interestingly, since only three of the five medical conditions are required for the diagnosis, it is possible to be of normal weight and still have the syndrome.

Stress. Yes, stress. This is complicated, and is probably due to the effects of chronic stress on hormonal activities in our brain. We know that stress increases cortisol levels (the "stress hormone"), which in turn raises glucose and insulin levels, increasing all the bad things they do. This may help to explain the connection between psychosocial stress and the development of heart disease.

Sedentary lifestyle. Just what you would expect. Less physical activity is directly related to heart attacks and strokes, as well as to the development of diabetes. Many components of the metabolic syndrome are clearly associated with an inactive lifestyle. These include a reduced HDL, increased blood pressure and blood sugar, and obesity. We'll consider what constitutes a sedentary lifestyle a little later and look at appropriate types, levels, and durations of various physical activities.

Aging. Not much to do about this, except to be aware that the incidence of this syndrome increases with increasing age. The number begins to approach one out of every two of us as we pass the fifty-year mark. And more women are afflicted with this than men.

Diabetes. In addition to being one of the defining factors of this disorder, it seems the syndrome itself increases the likelihood of developing type 2 diabetes. We're not sure which is the cart and which is the horse here, but the two are clearly connected. The same appears to be true for coronary heart disease.

So, we know the importance of this problem, how to diagnose it, and some of the things that cause it. Now, how do we fix it?

The cornerstone of treatment is a lifestyle evaluation and then appropriate change. Those changes will probably include increased exercise, a proper diet (a significant reduction in carbohydrate intake is important), adequate sleep, stress reduction (easier said than done), and targeted medication. This is a challenging issue to manage, and one that needs to be attacked on a multitude of fronts. While daunting, it can be done.

When it comes to medication, knowing where to start can be tricky, and it requires some expertise on the part of your healthcare provider. How we treat an irregular, complex laceration will help illustrate this point.

We see these types of wounds all too frequently in the ER and in our clinic. A child falls and busts his forehead; an elderly woman trips and strikes her forearm against the edge of a table, tearing her paper-thin skin in multiple directions; a teenager falls on his knee, bursting the skin over the kneecap. All of these wounds are difficult to repair. Where do you start? Nothing seems to fit together, and you wonder how you will ever be able to repair it. You take a deep breath, look at what you've got, and start with what you know goes where. One little piece at a time, properly placed and reattached. Then another, and another. Pretty soon, the puzzle starts to make sense, and somehow the jagged pieces come together. It's a great feeling for me, and a relief for my patient.

The same is true for dealing with the metabolic syndrome. We start with basic lifestyle changes, and then we begin to attack specific problems with carefully selected medications—one piece at a time. Pretty soon, the puzzle begins to make sense and things come together.

It takes a lot of work and effort on the part of the individual and a lot of support and guidance from their physician. But the results will be worth it—better control of their diabetes (maybe even eliminating the need for medication), better control of their blood pressure, better control of their weight, and less risk of a stroke or heart attack.

Who wouldn't want that?

18

Give Me the Details, Doc

HDL

Now let's talk about our "good cholesterol." Remember, though, HDL is not really a type of cholesterol. The HDL stands for "high density lipoprotein." It is another one of those entities that carries the cholesterol molecule through our bloodstream.

We are learning more about the function of HDL and its importance for maintaining a healthy lipid profile. But how does it exert a positive role and how has it come to be known as our "good cholesterol"?

This small particle is synthesized in the cells of the liver and small intestine. At first it contains no cholesterol but travels to various sites, including the walls of blood vessels, where it acquires free cholesterol molecules. Then it carries them to specific cells and tissues, as do the other lipoproteins. The difference is that HDL is a "reverse cholesterol transporter." While other lipoproteins are busy depositing their cholesterol in blood vessels and plaque, HDL is removing it from our system. This "reverse transportation" is obviously important and beneficial. It is one of the key steps involved in *reversing* cholesterol plaque size and reducing its instability—which are things we want to happen.

There has been a lot of discussion in the medical literature about HDL "particle size"—small versus large. This is not routinely measured and reported in your lipid profile, and probably not something your primary care physician routinely discusses with you. There's good reason for that. Some large studies have reported findings demonstrating that elevated amounts of "small HDL particles" are associated with increased reverse-transportation activity, and lower risk of developing cardiovascular disease. But other research indicates just the opposite. So right now, we just don't know. And until we've got this figured out, don't waste time on getting these additional studies done and don't waste time worrying about it. Again, we just don't know.

One thing we *do* know is that an elevated level of HDL is better than having a low level. Low levels (less than 40 mgs/dl in men and 50 in women) have been shown over and over again to be associated with the development of premature heart disease. By *premature* we mean heart disease in men before the age of fifty-five to sixty, and in women before the age of sixty-five. There is a clear connection between a low HDL and the occurrence of a first heart attack.

In addition, though we're not entirely sure why, low HDL levels are linked not only to the risk of a first major cardiovascular event (heart attack, stroke, sudden death), but also to the rate of all-cause-deaths. Put simply, if your HDL level is low, your chances are pretty good of something bad happening. And the lower your level, the higher your chances.

But just what causes low HDL levels? We've traditionally thought that poor diet and lack of exercise were major factors. While that still seems true, and correcting them remains a cornerstone of treatment, we are learning that genetic influences play a significant role. Some of these inherited problems have to do with a decreased formation of the HDL molecule, while some stem from an increased breakdown of the particle. We don't yet understand all the nuances here, but the potential is promising, and more information is being revealed every day. But remember, you can change your underwear, but you can't change your genes—at least not yet.

Now here's an interesting dilemma for patients and their healthcare providers alike: What do you do with a low HDL level but low or normal total cholesterol and LDL levels? In the past, we've generally not paid a lot of attention to this, pointing to a normal LDL level (the "bad cholesterol") and reassuring our patients that this, and not a low HDL level, is the main culprit.

Not so fast. We now know that an isolated low HDL is strongly associated with an increased risk of developing heart disease. For some reason, this is especially true in Asians. Since this represents a diverse but distinct genetic pool, it lends credence to the importance of genetic influences and puts more pressure on finding answers and effective treatments. By *effective*, we mean raising the HDL level and taking advantage of the molecule's protective effects on the development of atherosclerosis. But just what are those beneficial factors?

This is an area where we *do* know some things. First, the HDL molecule promotes the proper functioning of the endothelium, the cells that line the internal surfaces of our blood vessels. This is where the action is— where cholesterol plaques get started, grow, ulcerate, burst, and form clots. We want to keep our endothelium as healthy as possible.

HDL also prevents the oxidation of the LDL molecule—a key process in the development of those plaques. Unoxidized LDL is less likely to cause inflammation and disruption of our endothelial cell layer, hence the benefit of those antioxidants we constantly hear and read about.

Along with protecting against this oxidation of LDL, the HDL molecule helps prevent inflammation in the blood vessel wall, thus helping prevent the formation of plaque.

And finally, through a variety of actions and reactions, the HDL particle interferes with the clotting mechanism that represents the real danger of having an extensive cholesterol plaque. It's this clot that obstructs the blood vessel, depriving the tissues beyond it of needed oxygen and nutrients and leading to the heart attack or stroke.

We'll talk later about how to raise our HDL level, but for now, suffice it to say that the higher this number, the better.

What about a *really* high number? And what would that look like?

That's all part of the evidence that HDL helps protect against the development of heart disease and atherosclerosis. The higher the number, the less the incidence. And the magic number seems to be 75. Levels above that are associated with prolonged life—something called the "longevity syndrome." Again, there are probably genetic factors at play, but people with this level of HDL have much less incidence of coronary heart disease. That's interesting stuff, and something to keep in mind as we consider various interventions and treatments. But for now, remember that HDL is our friend.

19

Get Moving

We hear it all the time—

"Get up and do something!"

"Don't become a couch potato."

"Just do it."

We know we should be exercising, but sometimes it's hard to get started. Where do we find the motivation for that first step or first sit-up or first push-up? Maybe we need to start with the *why*, and then figure out the *how*.

It turns out the *why* is pretty overwhelming. The list of the benefits of physical activity is long and sometimes surprising.

As we would expect, exercise has a positive (protective) effect on the development of many common chronic conditions—heart disease, diabetes, chronic lung disease, kidney disease, and some kinds of cancers. Some experts believe the risk of recurrent breast cancer can be lowered by as much as 50 percent and the risk of developing colon cancer reduced by up to 60 percent. Alzheimer's disease falls into this category as well—something that should get the attention of those of us in our middle years and beyond. And it should come as no surprise that physical activity reduces the incidence of obesity, with all the problems associated with being overweight.

Now here are a few surprising benefits. The risk of osteoporosis is reduced with weight-bearing exercise. Bone mineral density increases, which reduces the possibility of a hip or other type of fracture. And since physical activity improves muscle tone and balance, the chances of falling are significantly diminished.

Exercise also decreases the risk of gallstones as well as improving brain function (again, lowering the risk of several types of dementia, including Alzheimer's). Regular physical activity can reduce stress and help lessen anxiety and depression. We previously mentioned that vigorous exercise can help you get to sleep faster and can improve the quality of your sleep, making it deeper and more efficient.

When it comes to lipids, the focus of this book, the benefits are important and straightforward. We know that regular exercise can lower LDL and triglyceride levels and raise HDL levels—all things we want to see happen.

With most of these benefits, the effect appears to be "dose-related"— the longer and more vigorous the exercise, the greater the improvements we experience in both physical and psychological well-being. But how much is enough, and what kinds of exercise are we talking about?

Without getting too complicated, it might be helpful to consider how exercise physiologists measure exercise levels. They use the term MET (metabolic equivalent) to compare various forms of physical activity. For instance, one MET equals the amount of oxygen an adult would consume while sitting at rest. *Moderate* physical activity (swimming, general house-cleaning, using a push mower, leisurely biking, and walking briskly at 3 to 5 miles per hour) would fall in the 3 to 6 METs range. *Vigorous* activity would be those things performed at greater than 6 METs, and include running, push-ups and pull-ups, and jumping rope (try *that* sometime if you really want a good workout).

So with those definitions in mind, what should be our goals? Here are a few suggestions and examples:

- Vigorous exercise of at least 20 minutes three times a week, combined with 30 minutes of moderate activity on most days, has been associated with a 50 percent reduced risk of death in men and women aged 50 to 71 years.

- Another option is to combine 150 minutes of moderate exercise with 75 minutes of vigorous exercise each week.

And for those of us who fall in the "overly compulsive" category, we can use METs to quantify our activity level. Solid experimental evidence indicates that expending 500 to 1,000 METs a week is necessary to achieve "substantial health benefits" (which these researchers define as a significant reduction in the risk of premature death and breast cancer). This equates to 150 minutes of walking each week (at 3.3 METs per minute, that gives you about 500). If so inclined, you can do the rest of the math to reach 1,000, combining various physical activities.

Measuring your heart rate, while sometimes helpful, is *not* necessary, thus saving us money on various monitors and contraptions. As we can see, the key factors are *time* and *intensity.*

"But Dr. Lesslie," someone might say, "I *am* a couch potato. Shouldn't I have my doctor check me over before I start an exercise program?"

That's a good question, and the answer is…maybe. But probably not. If you're in good health and don't have a history of a significant medical problem (heart disease, diabetes, uncontrolled high blood pressure), it's probably okay to get started. But do so gradually. Start slowly and build from there.

On the other hand, if you do fall into one of those categories, it will be a good idea to talk with your physician about how and when to begin. Be prepared though. If you ask ten doctors this question, you'll probably get eleven different answers.

If in doubt about the need for a medical evaluation before beginning a vigorous exercise program, you can find a helpful screening questionnaire at www.ncwc.edu/files/AHA.pdf.

The main point here is pretty simple—we need to get moving, and keep moving. Oh, and it's never too late to start.

20

You Gotta Know Your Numbers

The Eyes Have It

"Robert, I need some help with this one."

David Sasser, our newest and youngest ER doctor, walked up to the nurses' station and dropped the chart of room 3 onto the countertop. I was finishing up the record of a three-year-old boy in ortho. He had a fractured wrist, courtesy of his neighbor's trampoline—the orthopedist's best friend.

"Sure, Dave, what's the problem?"

I slid the three-year-old's chart to Amy Connors, our unit secretary. "Ortho consult."

She nodded, already dialing her phone—as usual, one step ahead of me.

"This fella, Russell Jenkins in room 3." Sasser rubbed his chin and studied the chart on the counter. "Nice guy. He works with Wells Fargo and handled the mortgage on our new house. He told me he was sitting at his desk this morning and lost vision in his left eye. Went completely blind—no pain or trauma or anything like that. Just happened out of the blue, and then he was back to normal. Only lasted ten seconds or so."

"What about now?" I glanced at Jenkins's ER record. Forty-six years old. Normal blood pressure and pulse. Normal visual exam. "Any headache or pain in his temple area?"

Pain or tenderness in this area can indicate the presence of inflammation in the temporal artery. If undiagnosed or untreated, it can lead to sudden and permanent vision loss.

"Nothing." Sasser shook his head and looked up at me. "He feels fine and has a completely normal exam. I was able to get a good look at his retina and it looks fine to me. If he'd been drinking or something like that, I wouldn't be so concerned. But he's a straight-up guy and he's worried. I just don't know what to tell him."

"Let's go see what we can find."

I grabbed the chart and we headed for room 3.

Russell Jenkins was sitting on the stretcher, arms propped on the edge of the thin mattress, studying his dangling legs. He looked up as I pulled the curtain closed behind us.

"Mr. Jenkins, I'm Dr. Lesslie. Dr. Sasser has told me about your vision loss this morning and I wanted to take a look."

"Sure, Doc. I just need to know what happened."

Sudden vision loss can be caused by a lot of things, none of which were good. But for his vision to return after a few seconds was something different, something unusual.

He repeated his story as I grabbed the opthalmoscope from its holder behind him. When I moved closer, I could see small yellowish raised areas just below his eyes. Xantholasmas—collections of cholesterol just below the skin. Common findings but unusual for someone his age.

"Do you take any medication, Mr. Jenkins? Blood pressure medicine or anything for an elevated cholesterol?"

"No, nothing. I've always been in good health and don't have any medical problems. But I have to admit, I keep pretty busy and haven't seen my family doctor in…four, maybe five years."

I was focusing the light on these golden, shiny areas, and David moved behind me, peering over my shoulder.

"I didn't see those," he whispered.

"See what?" Jenkins said, his eyes widening.

"Just these yellow areas below your eyes," I said. "Nothing serious, and they may not mean anything."

"They've been there awhile, but no one's ever said anything about them. My mother had the same things."

"Let's take a look at your eyes."

David switched off the overhead lights as I focused on the back of Mr. Jenkins's eye—the retina. The color was good and the optic disk was clearly visible, its edges clean and sharp. Everything looked fine, and I was pulling away when I saw it. And I froze.

At first I wasn't sure if it had been real. A faint glimmer—a golden reflection—had passed across his retina. It was small and streamed through one of his tiny arteries. Then it was gone, and I wondered if I had really seen anything at all. I waited a few seconds, and there was another one—gliding smoothly through one of his blood vessels.

I leaned back this time, and David flooded the room with a flick of the light switch.

"Everything okay, Doc?" Jenkins slumped back on the stretcher and rubbed his eyes.

"Let's take a listen to your neck." I was beside him now, placing my stethoscope over his left carotid artery. "Take a deep breath, then hold it."

Whoosh…whoosh…whoosh. The high-pitched noise, along with those yellowish deposits below his eyes, gave me the diagnosis. His carotid artery was clogged with cholesterol deposits, and the turbulence of blood flowing through this narrow pipe caused the whistling, whooshing sound. Small pieces of the plaque were breaking loose and finding their way to the artery that supplied his retina. A larger piece must have completely cut off blood flow momentarily, and then passed on through. The next time it happened, he might not be so lucky. Another piece might float to his brain and…

"Mr. Jenkins, we've got some work to do."

21

You Just Need to Calm Down: Stress and Your Cholesterol Level

You know the feeling—flushed face, heartbeat pounding in your ears, sweaty palms, breath catching in your throat. It's another "stress reaction"—your body responding to some real or perceived threat.

This is a normal reaction that God has equipped us with, and it is usually helpful. The old fight-or-flight response has saved many of us through the centuries. A giant grizzly bear appears out of nowhere, standing in front of us. Our brain responds in a split second. Adrenaline courses through our body, our heart rate speeds up, muscles tense, lungs work like mad, our GI tracts shut down (don't need that right now). Interestingly, we also experience a temporary reduction in our hearing as well as tunnel vision. We become focused on the threat in front of us. At the same time, cortisol (a hormone produced in our adrenal glands) floods our system, raising our blood pressure and driving up our glucose level. We're ready—our energy level boosted to warp speed—our muscles primed and waiting.

(Hmm...not going to be a fight this time. So it's flight, and we take off running, faster than we've ever moved before. Can't outrun a bear, though, so this might be a bad example.)

Anyway, this fight-or-flight response is a normal reaction, and though we're now quite "civilized," we still experience it regularly. While physical stressors and threats were the main factors in the past, our emotions now seem to be the prime culprits: anger, hate, challenge, fear, even love and joy.

All of these are intense feelings and can trigger a stress response. It might not be a bear in the woods, but how about that boss storming down the hallway to your office. Or those blue flashing lights in the rearview mirror. Or your mother-in-law appearing in your driveway for an unexpected visit. Face flushes, heart rate speeds up…you get the picture.

Fortunately, the response lasts only a few minutes, and then it gradually diminishes and disappears. The problem arises when this level of arousal becomes sustained—maybe not at the flushed-face level, but just beneath that intensity. Our heart rate remains a little above normal, we have a sense that our face is hot, though not beet-red, and there is an overall feeling of being on edge. These symptoms wax and wane but may never completely go away.

Now we're dealing with *chronic stress*, and that's *not* normal or in any way healthy. But it's all too common, and probably a product of our modern, highly "civilized" age. We are constantly bombarded and overloaded with information (the Internet, TV, radio, smartphones), conflicts (family, work, the national and international stages), and static (all the other things that grapple ceaselessly for our attention).

This heightened stress—hovering just below the fight-or-flight mode— does a lot of damage to our bodies, as well as to our spirits. We know that chronic stress is clearly connected to the development of diabetes, obesity, osteoporosis, and cardiovascular disease. In addition, we also know that this constant tension produces a heightened level of inflammatory markers in our bodies. This is associated with an increased incidence of rheumatoid arthritis, asthma, and various forms of dermatitis.

Just how does this happen, and what's the connection between chronic stress and our lipid levels? Let's go back for a moment to the fight-or-flight response. Remember, this is a natural and usually beneficial response. The chemicals and hormones released are designed to help us survive. It's when they remain at sustained levels that we start breaking down.

Let's first consider *adrenaline*, otherwise known as epinephrine. We've already mentioned its effects on our heart and cardiovascular system—an increased heart rate and elevated blood pressure. When this continues, problems develop. At the same time, adrenaline causes changes with our lipids. Free fatty acids are released into our bloodstreams, and over time, cholesterol and triglyceride levels become elevated. Adrenaline also causes a release of insulin, which further elevates our blood pressure, disrupts our normal lipid metabolism (by increasing cholesterol levels), promotes plaque formation in our arteries, signals our bodies to store fat, and when sustained, causes the cells in our body to become less and less responsive to its effects. This is the "insulin resistance" associated with the development of diabetes. It takes more and more insulin to do the same amount of work. Eventually, the cells in our pancreas that manufacture this hormone wear out and give up.

Elevated blood pressure, problems with insulin and glucose metabolism, and lipid abnormalities. This is beginning to sound like the *metabolic syndrome* again, isn't it? And that's exactly what's happening here. There is a real and significant connection between chronic stress and the metabolic syndrome, with all of its associated problems.

In fact, a recent and large study (more than ten thousand participants) compared workers who had little job-related stress with those who had significant levels of chronic stress. The researchers found that in the high-stress group, men had twice the risk of having the metabolic syndrome, while women had more than *five times* the risk.

But what about obesity? That's also part of this syndrome, right? That's where *cortisol*, the other stress hormone, comes into play. Though necessary and helpful in short bursts, when its levels remain elevated, it contributes to further elevations in our blood pressure, increased blood sugar (which leads to an increase in obesity), and impairment of our immune systems, with all the problems associated with that. Just think for a moment about family or friends (or maybe yourself) who have had to take prednisone for extended periods. What happens? They gain weight, their blood sugars get out of whack, and they are susceptible to a multitude of different infections. That's what cortisol does too.

Clearly, chronic stress takes a significant toll on our bodies. It's something we need to understand, to identify in our individual lives, and to eliminate as much as possible. Not an easy task, but it can be done.

The first step is to take a long, hard look at ourselves. For those brave enough, you'll find a questionnaire/diagnostic tool at http://healthscene investigation.com/files/2010/07/Percived-Stress-Scale.pdf that will help provide some insight and information. (And yes, the misspelling "percived" in the web address is correct.)

The treatment of chronic stress disorder is beyond the scope of this book, but the cornerstone of that treatment is based on lifestyle evaluation and appropriate change. Exercise, proper diet, adequate sleep, attention to our relationships and to our emotional and spiritual lives—it's all tied together.

This is really important, and it *can* be managed.

22

How'd Ya Sleep Last Night?

You might be wondering why I'm including a discussion about sleep in a book on cholesterol. Not very long ago, I would have wondered the same thing. But as we learn more about lipid disorders and about the harmful effects of inadequate sleep, we are faced with the reality that they are connected. In fact, sleep disorders seem to be connected with just about everything. And most of those things are pretty bad.

Since the most important and most prevalent sleep disorder is "obstructive sleep apnea," we'll save some time and ink and refer to this simply as OSA. So, just what do we know about OSA?

The Centers for Disease Control informs us that insufficient sleep is linked to the development of diabetes, cardiovascular disease (including high blood pressure, stroke, coronary artery disease, irregular heart rhythms such as atrial fibrillation, and hardening of the arteries), obesity, and depression. That's a long list, and should get our attention. Not only is OSA linked to these problems, but its presence makes the management of these disorders very difficult.

"Okay, Doc, but what's the connection between OSA and my elevated cholesterol level?"

The answer to that question has everything to do with something we've already looked at—the *metabolic syndrome*. OSA appears to be a significant contributor to developing this cluster of related problems. Remember, this is a group of disorders that includes abdominal obesity, difficulties with handling blood sugar, high blood pressure, and abnormal lipid levels. This last one is our concern here.

Mounting evidence connects OSA with a couple of lipid problems. The first has to do with HDL. The worse the OSA, the lower our good cholesterol. Second, the worse the OSA, the higher our triglyceride levels.

If these associations are real, you'd think that treatment of OSA would improve these abnormalities. It turns out that's just what happens. Adequate treatment results in a higher HDL, a lower triglyceride level, and even a lower total cholesterol level—all good things.

So we've established the connection between OSA and lipid problems. Now we need to know a little more about OSA, how the diagnosis is made, and what kinds of treatments are available.

Simply stated, OSA is a common sleep-related *breathing* disorder, marked by recurrent episodes of apnea (you stop breathing) and variable degrees of upper airway obstruction during sleep. Well, maybe not so simple. The bottom line is excessive daytime sleepiness, snoring, and gasping or choking during sleep. Think that might be you? No? Maybe you need to ask your spouse or roommate. Fortunately, several screening tests are available that should raise some red flags if you do have OSA.

The first and easiest to complete is the Sleep Apnea Clinical Score (SACS). It involves having someone measure the circumference of your neck. This is recorded in *centimeters* rather than inches because the smaller centimeter allows less error and variability in measurement. Then, the only things you need to know are whether you have high blood pressure (again, if you're on medication for this, you *have* high blood pressure) and whether you (1) snore or (2) have nighttime choking or gasping. With these factors, you simply utilize a chart and find your score. A number of 15 or above indicates a high risk of OSA. You can find a sample of this test at http://sleepmedicine.com/files/Forms/preoperative_questionnaire.pdf.

Another useful questionnaire is called the STOP BANG—an interesting acronym formed from the topics covered by the questions that are asked. It requires the following information:

Height in inches and centimeters: _____

Weight in pounds and kilograms: _____

Male/female: _____

Body Mass Index (BMI), which can be found in various tables, and you need to know your number: _____

Collar size of shirt: S, M, L, XL or _____ inches/cm

Neck circumference in centimeters: _____

With that information in hand, you simply answer a series of questions, which you can find at www.sleepapnea.org/assets/files/pdf/STOP-BANG%20Questionnaire.pdf. If you answer yes to three or more of these items, you're at high risk for OSA.

Lastly, you'll find the "Berlin Questionnaire" at www.sleepapnea.org/assets/files/pdf/Berlin%20Questionnaire.pdf. This is a little more involved, but will help answer the question of your personal risk for this problem.

"So what do I do if one or all of these tests indicate that I probably have OSA?"

If that's the case, it's time to sit down and talk with your doctor. The next step would be a sleep study, either done in your home (this is becoming much more acceptable and increasingly available) or in a formal sleep lab, where you'll need to spend the night. This will provide a definitive diagnosis and guide your healthcare provider in offering an appropriate treatment plan.

Several effective options exist, but a word of caution. Surgery used to be the go-to treatment for OSA, but it's painful, costly, and not always effective. I ask my patients who have had the procedure (easily determined by a routine exam of the mouth and throat) if they are happy with the outcome. Did it work and would they do it over again? Fewer than half (probably closer to one in four) have been helped by the surgery, and fewer still would do it again. If I had to make a decision for myself, I would quickly opt for a nonsurgical approach, such as a CPAP machine or an oral appliance (called a mandibular advancement device), both of which help keep a person's airway open while they sleep.

In the meantime, if you think you might suffer from OSA, here are some tips for improving your sleep. Actually, this is good advice for all of us.

1. Go to bed and get up the same time each day, even on weekends and holidays. Establish a rhythm.

2. Don't eat within three to four hours of going to bed. And don't overeat.

3. Limit caffeine and nicotine—none within three to four hours of going to bed.

4. Limit alcohol consumption in the same way. Remember that alcohol *interferes* with efficient sleep; it doesn't help it.

5. Establish a routine before turning off the lights, and stick to it. Take a shower or bath, read a book, listen to soothing music.

6. Avoid TV or computer games just before going to bed. Not surprisingly, it appears this stimulation also interferes with your sleep.

7. Create an environment conducive to restful sleep—cool, dark, quiet. Maybe consider a fan or other device to provide white noise to mask those bumps and thumps that might awaken you.

8. Quality pillows and mattresses (even sheets) are important and worth the investment.

9. Avoid long daytime naps—thirty minutes should be the max. Anything longer can make it harder to fall and stay asleep when you go to bed.

10. Regular physical exercise has been shown to help you fall asleep faster and to experience a deeper sleep. You'll need to experiment to determine how close to bedtime you can do this without being too energized.

For a lot of us, following these tips might be enough to help us sleep soundly and awake refreshed. For those who think they might have OSA, these will also be helpful, but you'll still need to complete a questionnaire, get tested, and find the best treatment plan for you.

Sweet dreams.

23

Water Is Our Friend

So, how long do you think you can live without food? If your answer is four to six weeks, you'd be right. Of course it all depends on a person's age and underlying general health, but a month to a month and a half seems to be about the limit.

How about water? Two days? Two weeks? Two months? The answer is about one week—not very long. Water is obviously very important to the human body, and provides as much as 60 percent of our total body weight.

But what else does water do for us? Water is important in the functions of digestion, circulation, transportation of important nutrients, temperature regulation, and the efficient performance of all our vital organs. Plain and simple—we just can't live without it.

Water does other things for us that might not be as obvious. Adequate hydration can keep your skin looking good—something important for a lot of us. And it helps with exercise and muscle functioning. Without adequate hydration, our muscles just don't work as well as they should. Our exercise workouts don't go as well as we want, and at the extreme, progressive weakness can lead to imbalance and dangerous falls.

When it comes to maintaining or losing weight, adequate water intake is essential. This works in a couple of ways. By substituting plain water for beverages that contain sugar or other sources of calories, we reduce our overall calorie intake. And drinking water before and with a meal has been demonstrated to reduce the amount of food consumed, thus contributing to weight loss.

This is what we're interested in when we're trying to control our lipid levels. Achieving and maintaining an ideal body weight moves us out of that metabolic syndrome tangle and into a much healthier state of being.

This is a good time to consider how what we've been learning all ties together. Previously, we considered the multiple benefits of physical activity. Exercise, especially *resistance training*, such as using free weights, builds muscle mass, which burns more calories, especially from fat stores, thus improving our lipid levels. Burning more calories reduces our weight, which lowers our blood pressure and improves our glucose levels.

But in the process, waste products are produced that need to be eliminated from our bodies. That's where our kidneys come in, doing what they do best—getting rid of these substances that we no longer need and that can cause damage when allowed to accumulate. That elimination takes water—enough to keep our kidneys flushing out these toxins.

That's the way God designed our bodies to work, and it all flows together, doesn't it? And it all requires an adequate amount of water.

But how much is enough? And what if I just don't like water?

Let's deal first with the "how much" part.

The old adage, "Make sure you drink eight glasses of water a day," probably still holds. But those need to be 8-ounce glasses. That amount correlates well with the current guidelines of about 3 quarts of liquid a day for men and a little less for women. I hope you noticed the word *liquid*. It doesn't all have to come from water, though that would be the easiest way of assuring an adequate intake. Other sources of liquid are other beverages as well as fruits and vegetables. Some of these contain a lot of water. So that helps answer the question about "not liking water." Each of us can find *something* we like to drink or eat.

This is another area where keeping a journal or log for a couple of weeks would be very helpful. Just record the amount of water and other beverages you consume daily, and see how it stacks up against that 3-quart goal. You'll probably be surprised. You just might not be getting as much as you think.

Keep in mind that amount is intended for *routine,* everyday life. If you're planning to engage in vigorous and prolonged exercise, you'll need to increase that goal. A hot, humid environment will also increase your needs, as will becoming sick. I remind my ill patients of the need to increase their fluid intake, and point out the vicious cycle that can quickly develop. We feel bad and don't drink enough water or other liquids. Then we become dehydrated, feel even worse, and drink even less. You get the picture. That's one of the times when we really need to pay attention to how much we're drinking.

For those other times, here are some tips for ensuring an adequate fluid intake:

1. Choose things to drink that you enjoy (just not with any sugar).

2. Drink something with every snack and especially with each meal.

3. Eat more fruits and vegetables. Remember, this is another good source of water, maybe as much as 15-20 percent of our daily needs.

4. Keep a bottle of water in your car or at your desk at work.

"But how will I know if I'm getting enough water each day?"

Even if you keep a log, you can count on your kidneys to provide this answer. If your urine is pale yellow and odorless, you're doing fine. If it's dark yellow and you notice a strong smell, you need to be drinking more. Keep in mind that our first morning urine is normally concentrated, so don't judge things by that.

"Is it possible to drink *too* much water?"

A medical school pathology instructor once told us that "anything can be a poison."

A fellow classmate who was awake and paying attention asked, "What about oxygen?"

"High concentrations of oxygen can cause permanent lung damage to newborn babies being cared for in a neonatal unit."

"Well, what about water?" the student persisted.

"Water intoxication is a well-defined entity, with the patient ingesting copious amounts of water, resulting in significant electrolyte derangements. Fortunately, it occurs only in patients with a psychiatric disorder, and only very rarely."

I can speak to the "very rarely" part. In almost forty years of practicing medicine, I've never had a patient get in trouble with drinking too much water. (I probably shouldn't have said that. After all, anything is possible.)

The bottom line here—adequate water intake is very important to our good health, and it is frequently overlooked. Make sure you're drinking enough.

Cheers!

24

Give Me the Details, Doc

LDL

As its name indicates, low-density lipoprotein (LDL) is another of our lipoproteins. It's larger than the HDL molecule, and is the "bad cholesterol" we talk about. It serves a purpose, though, and is essential to several key processes that are happening in various parts of your body as you read this page.

We mainly manufacture LDL in our liver but also in other organs and tissues. At present, we've discovered two patterns of LDL based on the size of the particle and determined largely by our genetics. Pattern A has larger, less dense LDL particles, while those of Pattern B are smaller and more compact. It's this latter Pattern B that's associated with a higher incidence of coronary heart disease, predicated on the assumption that the smaller molecules are better able to penetrate blood vessel walls and deposit their load of fat and cholesterol. Again, we're not completely sure about this, but growing evidence supports its validity, and it makes sense.

Under normal conditions, the LDL molecule does its important job of transporting various fats throughout the body, including fatty acids, triglycerides, and, of course, cholesterol. It is very efficient in this regard, and each molecule is able to carry as many as 1,500 particles of cholesterol through the blood and within the water surrounding our cells.

The problem occurs when the level of LDL in our blood becomes elevated, along with increased amounts of fats and cholesterol. That's when LDL transports and deposits these lipids into the walls of our arteries, attracting certain types of cells that begin the process of developing plaques in our blood vessels—atherosclerosis.

This is a good time to consider how this "hardening of the arteries" process gets started and progresses.

The first step is the development of a *fatty streak*. Unless you're related to the Tin Man, you've got some of these going on right now. We know from surgical cases and autopsies that this starts as early as childhood. In fact, one study of several thousand men and women between the ages of fifteen and thirty-four found *every* individual had these fatty deposits in their aortas.

These *streaks* are a thickening of the inside surface of the artery and are caused by the accumulation of a normally occurring cell, the *macrophage*. These are scavenger cells, cleaning up stuff that we don't need or want. They represent yet another example of how God has intricately designed our bodies. These cells have the unique ability of taking a single, specific amino acid—arginine—and converting it into nitric oxide, a "killer chemical," or into ornithine, a "repair molecule." If they make the nitric oxide, the macrophage is then able to ingest and destroy harmful things, such as bacteria. They are even able to do the same with some cancer cells. If they make ornithine, they are able to assist in wound healing, muscle repair, and other essential functions. Impressive.

When these macrophages are cleaning up excess lipids (deposited by our LDL molecules) they become overstuffed and are called "foam cells." Appetizing, isn't it? When enough of these foam cells accumulate, we have the beginning of a plaque in the inner layers of the artery—technically referred to as early *atheroma*. The veins of our body are constructed differently and don't develop these atheroma or any plaques.

As these areas expand, several things begin to happen. Smooth muscle cells move into places they don't belong, more macrophages are attracted, and more foam cells are formed. The plaque enlarges, and small blood vessels (capillaries) make their way through all of this, trying to supply blood to the artery wall. They can sometimes burst, bleeding into the plaque itself and causing sudden and sometimes deadly complications.

At this point, the plaque is composed mainly of fat, and as you would expect, it's relatively soft. That's why cardiologists are able to "balloon" these lesions, compressing them and placing a hollow tube or stent through the middle of it, allowing continued blood flow through the vessel.

If the plaque stays like this, and doesn't expand, it is said to be stable. It can remain in an artery for a long time and not cause any problems. It's when a plaque becomes unstable that things go wrong. This occurs when inflammation is present, and the plaque becomes "angry." Oxidized LDL molecules can trigger this response, causing those macrophages to release harmful chemicals that disrupt the stable plaque, leading to its ulceration and eventual rupture. That's when we have bleeding in the vessel wall and the formation of a blood clot, which can quickly enlarge and fill the entire artery. Then bad things happen: strokes, heart attacks, sudden death.

The process is more complex than this, but that's pretty much what happens. How and why that fatty streak gets started depends on multiple interconnected factors. Many things can affect the walls of our blood vessels, including high blood pressure, diabetes, smoking, and our individual genetic makeup.

And of course, abnormal lipids, of which LDL is the leading culprit, play a big part. That's why it's the "bad cholesterol." And that's why most experts now view attacking elevated levels of LDL as the most important part of dealing with abnormal lipids. It truly *is* the bad guy.

25

It's Okay to Go a Little Nuts

If you're like me and love almonds, walnuts, pistachios, and peanuts, this chapter will be nuttin' but good news.

You may remember a time when nuts of all varieties were considered unhealthy—too many calories and too much fat. I can remember my high school track coach admonishing us not to eat peanuts because it would "cut off our wind." I wasn't sure what that meant, but it sounded bad. And it took me until my third year of medical school to learn that peanuts were in fact not evil. I've always loved peanuts, and that was quite a relief.

It turns out the bad rap that nuts were given in the past was just that—a bad rap. Not based in any fact or science. Actually, we now know it's just the opposite. Nuts of just about all varieties are good for us. But how so?

Over the past ten years, a lot of research has been done on dietary habits and patterns. We've learned a lot, especially from the Nurses' Health Study. This is a group of more than 121,000 female nurses from eleven states. Coupled with that is a group of more than 50,000 male health professionals from all fifty states. These participants have been studied for more than thirty years—one of those topics being the effects of various diets. And one of these diet topics looked specifically at the relationship of nut consumption with several common and significant diseases. Their findings?

There is compelling evidence that frequently eating nuts can lower the incidence of heart disease, several types of cancer, cardiovascular disease, and diabetes. It is also associated with a reduction in death from these diseases, as well as several others. What makes this intriguing is that the more nuts consumed, the greater the impact on these positive findings. For instance, consuming 1 to 2 ounces of nuts *each day* results in the greatest reduction of these problems—much more so than once a week or not at all.

We also know that nuts can lower our levels of total cholesterol, triglycerides, and LDL, as well as raise levels of our HDL. Again, these changes are dose-related—the more consumed, the greater the impact.

But just which nuts are we talking about? Let's first consider the tree nuts, those we find…well, growing on trees. These are walnuts, almonds, pecans, and hazelnuts. Actually, hazelnuts (also known as *filberts*) grow on large bushes. I've got a dozen or so in my backyard, and these are peculiar critters. We can include pistachios, which grow on small trees and are closely related to the cashew. These are all probably interchangeable when it comes to nutritive value and the positive impacts on our health. And they will all have the beneficial effects on our lipids that we're interested in. You may have heard or read that walnuts, as well as almonds, stand out in this group. The reality is that *all* of these nuts are good for us.

"But what about cashews and Macadamia nuts? And I love Brazil nuts. What about all of those?"

These nuts also confer positive effects on our lipids, as well as lowering the incidence of the diseases mentioned above. The problem is the amount of fat and calories they contain. Nuts are calorie and nutrient dense, and these nuts are *super* dense. While not bad for you, you've got to really be careful about the amount you eat—something I'm not very good at.

You might be thinking, "What about peanuts?" You're right. We haven't included the lowly peanut in any of these lists. And for good reason.

My college biology professor would quickly point out that the peanut is *not* a nut but a *legume*—same family as beans, peas, and lentils. Yet we call them nuts. So how do they stack up against the tree nuts? This is important, since we eat many more peanuts than we do almonds or walnuts or pecans.

Well, I told you this chapter would be all about good news. It turns out that peanuts provide all the same benefits as our tree-nut friends. This includes lower rates of mortality, less heart disease and cancer, lower triglyceride and LDL levels, and increased HDL levels.

There's something else here of interest. We're all aware of the studies that suggest that drinking a glass of red wine each day is good for your heart and that it can help prevent the development of plaques in our arteries. That's probably due to the presence of *resveratrol*, a potent antioxidant. And guess what—there's more resveratrol in peanuts than in red wine. That's in addition to high levels of vitamin B_3 (niacin), which we use to lower our triglycerides and raise our HDL level. This is all good news to me.

Clearly, we need to be including nuts in our daily diets. But how much is enough? Or too much? The guidelines now indicate 1 to 1.5 ounces a day—about a good handful. Twice that amount might even be better, but you have to keep track of your total caloric intake. Remember, nuts of all varieties are nutrient dense—loaded with good stuff but also with calories.

Here are some pointers:

- Incorporate nuts into your diet by *replacing* something else, not just adding them on.

- Nuts make a great snack, and because of their high protein content, will gradually release their energy, helping us control those late-morning and afternoon hunger attacks.

- It doesn't matter whether nuts are roasted. This process changes the flavor but not the nutritional value.

- It probably *does* matter about added salt and cooking oils. This can be a problem for those of us with high blood pressure or who need to lose weight.

- Eat a variety (unless you're allergic to peanuts) and do so every day.

- You can include peanut butter in this mix. Just be sure to read the label, paying special attention to the carbohydrate content and the list of ingredients. "All natural" and "organic" might be preferred, but read that label.

There's one more point about nuts that we need to consider, something that has posed a significant dilemma for quite a while. Is the correct pronunciation *pea'-con* or *pea-con'* or *pea'-cun* or *pea'-can* or *pea-can'*? I'm from the South, and will stick with *pea-can'*. Ya'll will have to decide for yourselves.

26

When Lifestyle Changes Just Aren't Enough

"Dr. Lesslie, I think I messed up."

Lori carefully slid two charts on the counter beside me. I glanced at the one closest and saw the name—Dave Jernigan.

"Good. Dave and Lisa are back to check on their lipids. Why do you think you messed things up?"

Lori flipped open Dave's chart. A copy of his most recent lab work stared up at me. The lab company who provided the reports did us a favor—anything out of whack was printed in bold numbers. There were a lot of bold numbers on Dave's sheet.

"I gave the Jernigans their copies and heard Mr. Jernigan explode right after I closed the exam room door. Good luck."

She scooted down the hallway and disappeared.

I thumbed through his record, searching for the lipid panel we had done on his previous visit. That was three months ago, and things should have improved by now.

Not.

Dave's total cholesterol had started at 289. Today it was 284. And his LDL hadn't budged either. It had been 160 on his first visit and was 161 now. Fortunately, his triglycerides were good—still under 150—and his HDL was essentially the same at 41 compared to 39 before. *He's not going to be happy about this.*

Lisa's labs were a little better. Her total cholesterol, LDL, and HDL were still normal, and her triglycerides, which had been elevated at 279, were now 175. Moving in the right direction, but we weren't quite where we needed to be.

I had barely closed the door behind me when Dave exclaimed, "Alright, Dr. Lesslie, I did everything you told me to do, and nothing happened. Explain that."

His face was flushed and he leaned forward on the exam table, the copy of his lab report clutched in his hand. Lisa sat quietly in the corner of the room.

"I've been exercising like crazy—thirty to forty minutes every day on the treadmill. I've cut way down on sugar—haven't I, honey?"

Lisa nodded and smiled.

"No more sweetened iced tea," he continued. "We haven't had any beef in…at least a month. And with that Mediterranean Diet, I feel like I've got fruit and olive oil coming out of my ears. I don't get it. What else am I supposed to do?"

"There *is* some good news here, Dave. You've lost almost five pounds, and that's not easy. So you're doing something right. And Lisa, you've lost a couple of pounds too."

"Her triglycerides are a lot better now," Dave said, "so this is working for her. But I'm dead in the water. Nothing's happening. I might as well be eating cheeseburgers and french fries."

Our eyes met and his long, loud sigh filled the room. He leaned back against the wall.

"What now?"

I rolled the exam stool toward me and sat down.

"You're working hard, Dave, that's why you've lost some weight. Sometimes, though, the things you've been doing just aren't enough, no matter how hard you try. I think it's time to consider some medication."

He glanced at Lisa and sighed once more.

"I know you're not wild about the idea," I told him. "But we've got some good choices, and I think three months from now you're going to see some big changes."

"*Something's* got to change, Doc. Tell me what we're talking about here."

27

You Gotta Know Your Numbers

Tick...Tick...Tick

Sam Wiggins came through the triage door in a wheelchair.

"Another kidney stone, Doc." The sixty-four-year-old shook his head and beads of sweat dropped to his lap. "This one's a doozy."

Lori Davidson pushed him past the nurses' station and into room 5. She turned to me and said, "I'll get a urine sample as soon as we can," then pulled the curtain closed behind them.

I glanced at the chart of room 1 and finished making my notes on the forty-two-year-old with pneumonia.

"We'll need a chest X-ray and some blood work, Amy. And I think his wife is out in the waiting room. She might want to come back now."

Amy reached for the chart and picked up her phone. "Looks like Sam has another kidney stone." She tilted her head toward room 5.

Both Amy and I had seen Sam on at least a half dozen occasions looking just like this—pale, sweating, and pacing up and down the hall.

Pacing. He usually walked into the ER and wouldn't sit down. Typical for people with stones. They try without success to move around and find a comfortable position. But not this time. Sam had been sitting rigidly in that wheelchair, white-knuckling the armrests. Something—

"Dr. Lesslie, this is Mrs. Masters, the wife of the man in room 1," Amy said. She motioned behind me with her head, and I turned around.

"Mrs. Masters, I'm Dr. Lesslie. Let me tell you about your husband, and then we can head on into his room. First though, he's going to be alright."

I explained what was going on and what we would be doing, and I was about to take her to her husband when the emergency room doors burst open. Several EMTs raced into the department with two teenagers on a pair of emergency medical service stretchers. I quickly learned they had been involved in an auto accident on Highway 21. It was a bad wreck, and the next hour was occupied with getting them stabilized.

One of the injured young men was being wheeled down the hall to the operating room, and the other had just left by helicopter, headed toward the trauma center in Charlotte. Lori was standing at the nurses' station, and I walked to her side. She was studying Sam Wiggins's chart and shaking her head.

"Has he gotten some relief from his pain?" I glanced at the urinalysis report, noting the large amount of blood. "Looks like he *does* have another stone."

Bret Jones, one of the other ER doctors on duty, had been taking care of Sam while I had been in Trauma. It had been a while, and Wiggins should be better by now.

"He's still in a good bit of pain," Lori answered. "But he won't complain about it. Dr. Jones checked on him a little while ago, and Sam told him he was okay. But he's just lying on the stretcher, holding his sides and not moving."

Where was the pacing? If this was a stone and he was still in pain, he'd be up and moving around the room, not lying motionless.

"It sure acts like a kidney stone, Dr. Lesslie," Lori said. "But something's not right. His heart rate keeps going up—and I know that can be his pain. But his blood pressure is starting to fall a little."

An alarm exploded in my head.

"What's a little?"

I dropped the clipboard for Trauma and hustled around the nurses' station, headed for room 5.

"It's one ten over seventy, but his blood pressure has always been a little high every time he comes in."

Lori was right. Sam Wiggins had problems with his blood pressure, and wasn't convinced he needed to take his medication regularly. A pressure of 110/70 might be a little low for most men his age and size, but for Sam it was really low.

I pulled the curtain open. Sam's wife was dabbing his forehead with a wet paper towel and looked up at me. I didn't take my eyes off her husband. He was damp with sweat, and his color was as white as the sheets of his stretcher.

I hurried to the side of his bed and pulled the sheet away from his abdomen.

"Tell me about your pain, Sam."

He was listless now and having trouble focusing. He tried to point to some area of his belly, but his hands flopped to the stretcher.

"Tell me about any medical problems Sam has," I said to his wife, who was standing just behind me now. "I know about his hypertension, but is there anything else? Any other medication?"

Sam's abdomen was tense now, and my palpations caused him to moan quietly.

"Ninety over fifty." Lori was on the other side of the stretcher and her tone got my attention.

"Just the kidney stones," his wife answered. "But you already know about that. And his cholesterol. He's always had trouble with it, but he won't take the medicine his doctor gave him. He says it causes leg cramps. His doctor says it's really high and has tried different things, but Sam won't take any of it. I've told him—"

I was searching for a pulse over his right femoral artery. Nothing. And nothing on the left.

"Eighty over forty."

I leaned close to Lori. "Have Amy call the OR supervisor stat. And get whoever's on for vascular surgery on the phone. This isn't a kidney stone. Sam has an aortic aneurysm, and if it hasn't blown, it's just about to."

Lori rushed out of the room and over to our secretary.

I turned to Sam's wife. "Mrs. Wiggins, let me tell you what's happening here."

A bedside ultrasound confirmed the diagnosis. Sam's aorta was ballooning, but there wasn't any free blood—not yet. The walls of the blood vessel were calcified, weakened by layers of cholesterol deposits. This hadn't happened overnight.

Later that evening, the vascular surgeon came by the ER and told us about Sam's operation.

"We were minutes from losing him, Robert. That thing was seconds away from rupturing. But he made it through the surgery, and he's okay— for now."

Chapter 28

When All Else Fails...
and You Need a Pill

One of our goals as healthcare providers should be to limit the need and use of medications as much as possible. We also understand that's the hope of most of our patients. With some medications and conditions, that won't be possible. The person with type 1 diabetes will always need insulin. And someone with a surgically absent or nonfunctioning thyroid gland will forever need thyroid hormone replacement.

With lipids disorders, there is the distinct possibility of tapering or one day eliminating the need for medications. This will depend on effective and permanent improvement in lifestyle issues—something that in my experience doesn't happen very often.

That leaves us with the need for medications that will help us get the job done, just as in Dave Jernigan's case. Fortunately for Dave, and the rest of us, we have a growing array of options. We'll briefly consider these, and then take a more comprehensive look at those most commonly used.

The most important and most commonly prescribed are *statins*—technically the HMG-CoA reductase inhibitors. We refer to them as statins because these drugs all end with...that's right, "statin." Pravastatin, simvastatin, atorvastatin. And also because it's easier to say "statin" than the technical name. The discovery of the statins has proved to be a significant milestone in the treatment of lipid disorders. There are a few side effects we need to consider, but statins have emerged as the first line of treatment for an elevated cholesterol or LDL level, and should be the first prescription your physician writes if you need medication.

Another class of drugs frequently used for this disorder is the *fibrates*. This includes fenofibrate (Tricor), gimfibrozil (Lopid), and a few other newer medications. They are almost always used in conjunction with a statin (unless those drugs aren't tolerated), and their main effects are to lower serum triglyceride levels and raise HDL levels. They accomplish these beneficial actions through several mechanisms, including reduced secretion of VLDL from the liver (see chapter 45) and by directly stimulating the manufacture of HDL. They are expensive, and some questions remain as to their long-term impact on cardiovascular health and outcomes.

The *bile-acid sequestrants* are another group of drugs that act in an entirely different manner. They bind bile acids in the intestines, which results in a significant reduction in their reabsorption. When this happens, the amount of available cholesterol diminishes, and we see lower levels of cholesterol and LDL. These are the main benefits, with only a slight elevation sometimes noted with our HDL. Drugs in this class include cholestyramine, colestipol (Colestid), and colesevelam (Welchol). Since they act in the GI tract, that's where we see most of their side effects—constipation, nausea, upset stomach.

Another and newer class of medication is the *cholesterol absorption inhibitors*, and they do just that. They also act in the GI tract and directly block the absorption of cholesterol. The main drug here is ezetimibe (Zetia) and some studies demonstrate that it can lower LDL by 15 to 17 percent. It's also expensive, and though well-tolerated, the jury is still out as to its long-term effectiveness and where it fits in our efforts to make a real difference with abnormal lipid levels.

These are the main choices we have, as far as prescription drug classes go. The key is to match the right medication with the individual and their specific needs. Then it becomes a matter of trial and error (hopefully not much error). If you've been on any of these drugs, you know it may take awhile to find the right one(s) and the correct dosages.

There will be a solution here, something that will help us get this problem under control. But it's critical to remember those lifestyle changes we've discussed. Taking a pill doesn't erase the need for a proper diet or exercise or any of those other things. Lipid disorders are multilayered and require a multipronged approach.

29

The Statins

The discovery of the statin drugs was a major breakthrough in the treatment and prevention of elevated cholesterol levels and its related diseases. But this didn't happen out of the clear blue and certainly not overnight.

It began in the early 1970s with the work of a Japanese biochemist, Akira Endo. He was searching for an enzyme that would be useful in the beverage industry—removing impurities encountered in the production of wine and ciders. Later, his work involved a fungus in the *Penicillium* family. (Sound familiar? What about Alexander Fleming and the discovery of penicillin?) Endo was trying to find something that would inhibit the synthesis of cholesterol, and came upon two such compounds. One (he called it ML-236B) later came to be known as mevastatin, the precursor of our first statin drug, lovastatin.

Several years would pass before the pharmaceutical giant Merck would develop and market this new drug, also known as Mevacor. And the statin industry exploded.

Prior to this new class of medicine, the medical and scientific world knew the harmful effects cholesterol caused to our blood vessels and hearts. Several anticholesterol drugs were on the market, but all had bothersome side effects, including gastrointestinal discomfort, flushing, liver disease, and the formation of gallstones. Lovastatin, with its effectiveness and rare side effects, was a welcomed addition to our battle against cholesterol and heart disease.

Have the statins lived up to their hype and proved helpful? The answer is an overwhelming yes. While cardiovascular disease and strokes remain significant problems, over the past thirty years we have experienced a 50 percent reduction in deaths due to these diseases. Several factors are responsible for this, but the emergence of statin therapy appears to be a major contributor.

How do these drugs work and what do they do?

Remember that the formation of the cholesterol molecule is a thirty-seven step process. All of the statin drugs block the action of HMG-CoA, a rate-limiting enzyme critical to cholesterol synthesis. "Rate-limiting" means that if you can block this early step, you can stop the ultimate manufacture of cholesterol. And that's what happens.

There are multiple statin drugs now, each with its own potency and safety profile, but each acts in this same way. They block the action of this rate-limiting enzyme, and they do this mainly in the liver.

Okay, that's how they work, but what good do they do for us? We know that the statins are the most powerful drugs available for lowering LDL levels—somewhere in the range of 30 to 60 percent. They can slightly raise HDL levels by 5 to 10 percent—a modest difference but still helpful. And they can lower triglycerides anywhere from 20 to 40 percent.

All of these are important factors in the prevention and management of the many cardiovascular diseases that afflict us. We already mentioned the reduction in deaths, and this is brought about through several mechanisms. First, the plaques that plague each of us are stabilized—less growth and inflammation. The underlying damage to our vessel walls is reduced and possibly reversed. This makes it less likely that clotting will take place, which we know is what ultimately blocks critical arteries and causes the heart attacks and strokes we're trying to prevent.

All of this is important, and the statins are effective weapons in this struggle. In the next few chapters we'll consider some of their other benefits as well as some of their problems. And if you need one of these drugs, we'll take a look at determining which one will be right for you.

30

The Other Benefits of Statins

We need to have a good understanding of how medical studies are performed, and then use that understanding to determine how we should respond to the constant barrage of new health claims and "breakthroughs." We'll look at that in depth in another chapter, but here's a thumbnail sketch of things to keep in mind.

The "latest studies" and "recent research" usually represent only the first steps in a process of validation—determining if the breakthroughs or findings are real. We live in an age of instant—no, *micro*-instant—communication, and with a media whose task it is to forever whet our appetites for something exciting, new, and different. In the vernacular of the Old West, we "fire from the hip" and frequently fail to take careful aim. Half-baked evidence is presented as irrefutable fact, and inadequately scrutinized research is proclaimed as the Gospel. New cures for cancer, the diabetic drug that promises miraculous relief, the newly discovered benefits of a familiar food. All too often it's only a flash in the pan. A lot of excitement, then nothing—and we're on to the next biggest thing.

This can be difficult to guard against, but if we keep a couple of things in mind, we will be able to sit back and wait for the final verdict. This is where the types of medical research come into play.

Here's what happens. A researcher or scientist notices something unexpected. It might have to do with a drug, or a treatment, or a phase of the moon. She suspects an association—some important piece of information that might come from what she has observed.

Let's take the moon as an example. The researcher notices one night that when the moon is full, the labor and delivery unit of the local hospital is full to overflowing. She decides to examine the hospital records, comparing dates of birth with the phases of the moon. This is an "observational" type of study, and it's the easiest to perform. For a variety of reasons, it also gives the least accurate information. Lo and behold, for the previous six months, more births occurred during the days around a full moon than at other times. The researcher reports this finding, a newspaper picks it up, and everyone gets excited. Pretty soon, it becomes a "known fact."

Only later do we learn the real truth. Larger and more objective studies fail to demonstrate the association between a full moon and an increase in newborns, yet the "known fact" persists. (And no, there is no conclusive evidence that the full moon is connected with women giving birth. The only solid association we have with this lunar phenomena is the assured appearance of werewolves.)

The same sort of thing happens with new medications. A beneficial effect is noticed with a certain type of medication, usually through an observational type of study, and the association is presented as fact. The passage of time and further, more objective studies might bear this out. Or they might not. The beneficial effect wasn't real, or wasn't significant, or in the worst case, actual harm might have been done.

That was the case with thalidomide in the late 1950s. This was a "wonder drug," a magical cure for anxiety and insomnia. When found to alleviate morning sickness, it was given to thousands of pregnant women. The results were devastating, with tragic birth defects afflicting tens of thousands of newborns. The drug was yanked from the market, but not before the damage was done. More recently, we were faced with the fen-phen problem. This combination of medicines was a very effective weight-loss drug. It worked, and a lot of people were taking it. And a lot of people developed a specific and serious heart problem. It was yanked from the market as well.

The problems with these drugs were multiple—not enough research, not enough animal trials, not enough time. We greeted them with open and trusting arms, and we paid a big price. This is not ancient history, and some of the same problems exist today. All too frequently we read articles about the unexpected problems with highly touted medications, usually attached with the names of ever-available attorneys.

But what does any of this have to do with "the other benefits of statins"? Actually, a lot. I'm going to present information here, some of which is grounded in solid research (the most accurate coming from multiple randomized trials). Some of this you may have heard about, and I'll give you the latest on where that information stands. Some of these associations will come from observational studies—interesting, hope-inspiring, but not yet established as something we can count on. That will take more time and research.

So what are some of these things we know or think we know about statins?

Let's start with cancer—something we all would like to see eradicated from this earth. Several observational studies have previously raised the possibility that statins may decrease the overall risk of certain types of cancer. While this has captured the attention of the media and most physicians (myself included), large studies have not been able to substantiate this link. At this time, there is no solid evidence to support these initial findings. Fortunately, these same large studies did *not* identify any risk of the statins causing cancer.

The evidence regarding dementia is more compelling. Statins appear to decrease the risk of several kinds of dementia (including Alzheimer's) and to possibly slow its progress. Good news for all of us.

There's also good news for those of us with kidney disease. Statins appear to be able to preserve renal function in the face of chronic disease, as well as being protective for those whose kidneys are normal.

The evidence is not so good when it comes to multiple sclerosis. A year or so ago there was some hope that statins might be able to reduce the risk of developing this dreaded disease. To date, large randomized trials have not been able to demonstrate this effect. The jury may still be out on this one, but the door appears to be closing.

There are other areas where the evidence is solid for a beneficial impact of these drugs. Statins may decrease the risk of venous blood clots, lower blood pressure in those with hypertension, improve outcomes in individuals with heart failure, and protect and preserve our bones—reducing osteoporotic fractures. Lastly, these drugs appear to reduce the incidence of pancreatitis and the risk of needing surgery for those of us with gallstones. All of this is good news. Again, time will bring clarity and hope-fully more good news.

Meanwhile, my advice is to remain cautiously optimistic. And if it weren't bad for your blood pressure, I'd suggest taking most of the bally-hooed breakthroughs with a grain of salt.

Statins: The Downside

In spite of all the benefits of the statin drugs, there is a real downside and some problems we need to be aware of. You've heard or maybe experienced the muscle pain associated with these medicines, and we'll look at that. But first, let's consider some of the other possible side effects.

Serious problems with statins occur very rarely, only in a very small percentage of people taking them. And we need to understand that problems occur less frequently with statins than with other classes of lipid-lowering drugs. Here's what we know.

Since these medications are metabolized in the liver, there is a possibility of damage to this organ. This is rare and usually manifests as an elevation in our liver enzymes, without any symptoms—hence the need to check these enzyme values before starting one of the statins. There has been an ongoing debate as to how often these lab tests need to be repeated. The FDA currently advises that repeat studies need be done only if there is some clinical reason to do so, such as fatigue, weakness, or muscle pains. It's not unreasonable to repeat this liver panel once, usually around three to six months after starting the drug, and to monitor for any symptoms beyond that.

Some troubling information exists that the statins might influence the onset of diabetes in those previously nondiabetic but with a predisposition. The evidence here is conflicting. It appears that if this is real, its impact is very small, and it usually occurs with those people who are receiving high levels of the medication.

Some evidence exists that these drugs may be associated with the development of certain types of cataracts.

While there have been concerns about the development of kidney problems while on statins, recent large studies have failed to establish any association.

Likewise, there has been concern about these drugs and an increased incidence of various cancers. And as with possible kidney problems, no clear association has been proven.

For patients who are pregnant or trying to become so, the recommendation is to stop or don't start these medications. There is no solid evidence that statins are harmful to the fetus; if they are, the effects appear to be very small. But why take the chance?

Now let's consider those muscle pains. After all, this is what causes the most problems for our patients and is what brings them back to the office.

Let's start with some definitions. *Myalgia* is the term used for muscle aches, tenderness, soreness, and cramps. These cramps can occur during or after exercise. It's the least serious of our muscle problems and is not associated with a rise in one of our muscle enzymes—creatine kinase (CK)—used for diagnosing muscle disease or injury. A *myopathy* is a muscle weakness and can be a painful condition. It may or may not occur with an elevation of the CK level. *Myositis* is inflammation of the muscle, and almost always is found with an elevated CK and associated pain or tenderness.

When we talk about muscle problems with the statins, we're usually dealing with myalgia—aches and soreness. This occurs in as many as 2 to 11 percent of people taking these drugs, and when mild, frequently goes away after a few weeks of treatment. The more severe forms of muscle damage (myopathy and myositis) happen much less often—in less than one tenth of one percent of individuals.

At this point, we're not sure how statins cause these problems, but we do know statins are inhibitors of HMG-CoA in the liver—an enzyme also found in our muscles. Once we know exactly what's going on here, we should be able to prevent and treat this bothersome side effect.

We *do* know who may be at risk of developing muscle problems, and it starts with the specific statin drug itself. The risk appears to vary among the different drugs, with pravastatin (Pravachol) and fluvastatin (Lescol) having the lowest incidence of myalgia and myopathy. (They are also our least potent statins.) The other drugs in this class have variable and higher risks than these two, especially at higher doses. Individuals with preexisting muscular problems are at higher risk, including those with amyotrophic lateral sclerosis (ALS) and genetically based muscle diseases. We also know that hypothyroidism (undiagnosed or inadequately treated) is another risk factor, as is a low blood level of vitamin D.

One of the biggest areas of concern involves the interaction of statins with other drugs, including prescription, over-the-counter, and herbal medicines. We previously considered that many of us do not share our use of herbal products with our physician, and this can lead to serious complications.

The most common and potentially most dangerous interaction has to do with how various drugs are metabolized. Many of the statins are broken down by a specific enzyme system, and a number of drugs inhibit this system, causing it to be inactive. The statins then remain active in our system, and their concentrations can rise to significant and harmful levels. A list of these drugs is long, but here are some common and familiar examples:

- amlodipine (Norvasc)
- cimetidine (Tagamet)
- ciprofloxacin (Cipro)
- erythromycin
- metronidazole (Flagyl)
- clarithromycin (Biaxin)
- ketoconazole (an antifungal medicine)
- several medications for the treatment of HIV
- tetracycline

Other medications that can increase the risk of muscle problems include the fibrates (another class of lipid-lowering medications) and possibly niacin, though the evidence here is mixed.

This is probably a good time to mention statins and grapefruit juice. Conventional wisdom has previously informed us that you should never eat grapefruit or drink its juice while taking a statin, since grapefruit can inhibit this same enzyme system. That's no longer the accepted wisdom.

Adequate data exist demonstrating that up to eight ounces of juice or one-half a grapefruit is fine and won't affect your statin levels.

Something else that probably needs to be debunked is the concern that regular physical exercise might place your muscles at risk. This doesn't appear to be the case either.

The issue of muscle soreness and cramps can sometimes prove perplexing. We are physical creatures and our muscles just ache sometimes. And we get the flu, with its muscle pains. So how do we make the diagnosis of statin-induced myalgia or myopathy?

First, you need to be taking one of these drugs. (You won't have to go to medical school to figure that one out.) And then you'll need to answer a few questions.

When did the symptoms start? The onset is usually within a few weeks to months after starting the medicine, with an average of a little over six months.

Where do your muscles hurt? Statin related pain typically starts in our proximal muscles, those closest to our core—upper arms and thighs. And this usually occurs in a symmetric fashion, meaning that both arms or both legs are affected.

What about weakness or any physical impairment? Frequently we'll see patients who have difficulty climbing stairs, raising hands above their head, or getting up from a chair. They may also complain of cramping, especially at night. (Again, there are several things besides statins that can cause this.)

What about blood work? We mentioned CK, a specific muscle enzyme that is released when muscle fibers are damaged. This may or may not be present, so its elevation helps establish the diagnosis, but a normal level doesn't rule it out.

Okay, let's say we have a diagnosis of statin-induced myopathy, now what?

If we're sure of the diagnosis, it's time to stop the medication. Symptoms should resolve over the next few weeks, and in the vast majority of instances, no long-term damage is done. We'll recommend plenty of water intake and maybe some localized heat. Other than that, there's no specific treatment needed or available.

What if you have a muscle problem with a statin, but you really need to be on one? You have elevated lipids and proven heart disease.

That poses a dilemma, but not one that will be insurmountable.

The first step is to check for any potential drug interactions. This includes those herbal remedies you didn't tell your doctor about. Then we need to check on your thyroid. If you're on thyroid hormone replacement medication, the correctness of the dose needs to be determined. This changes over time, and you'll never know unless you have it tested. Finally, we need to know the level of your vitamin D. As we discussed previously, as many as three out of every four people we test in our clinic have low levels. This is easily fixed.

If at this point nothing turns up, it's reasonable to consider restarting one of the statins—preferably pravastatin or fluvastatin, since they pose the least risk of causing a myopathy. And if that's not effective, we can try every-other-day dosing, or even less frequently.

It should be stressed that in the very rare instance of a severe muscle problem (extensive tissue breakdown, kidney problems, and hospitalization), statins should never, ever be used again.

The bottom line here is that many of us need statin medication, and the vast majority of those who do will tolerate at least one of the statin drugs without any problems. If you're taking a statin, make sure you know what side effects to look for and talk with your physician if you develop any of these symptoms.

Thankfully, this is one of those times when the benefits clearly outweigh any potential risks.

32

Hot Off the Press

As I write this, the American Heart Association is concluding its annual meeting in Chicago. A Scottish researcher presented a fascinating study there, dealing with the very issues we have been considering, and the report is both exciting and challenging.

First the *exciting part*: Taking a statin drug for as little as five years during middle life (in this study, forty-five to sixty-four years of age) resulted in fewer heart attacks and less heart failure, and it also reduced the chances of dying from *any* cause. The numbers are impressive—a 35 percent reduction in heart attacks and death. This was determined after the end of the five years of treatment. (The study began in 1989.)

That's good news, and confirms the results of a multitude of other studies. What makes this study stand out is that these results—the reductions in heart attacks and death—persisted, even after study participants stopped taking the medication at the end of the study. Twenty years later, the researchers found a 27 percent decrease of heart attacks in these individuals when compared to others never having taken a statin drug, and a 13 percent reduction in overall deaths. They conclude that these benefits extend for decades, and may in fact grow and include some of the other positive findings we've previously considered.

Those are amazing findings, and if substantiated by further studies, will shake the foundations of the preventive medicine world.

The *challenging part*: Identifying those individuals who will benefit most by taking these medications. This study included some people with evidence of early heart disease, but others with an elevated LDL level and clean arteries. Everyone seemed to be helped, and that might be the answer. A low-dose statin might become as commonplace as taking a baby aspirin each day.

Other challenges remain. What will turn out to be the best dose? How do we effectively prevent muscle pain and damage? How do we make sure this treatment is accessible and affordable? How do we get the word out to those of us in the trenches of primary care?

As with any "hot off the press" study, these results will need to be taken apart and looked at closely. While this report included more than six thousand individuals, larger trials will need to be conducted to confirm—hopefully not refute—these findings.

In the meantime, if you're like me and currently taking a statin, this is one more encouraging piece of information.

33

Which Statin Is Best for Me?

We now know the benefits and possible side effects of the statin drugs. If your physician recommends that you begin taking one of these, and you're convinced of the need to do so, this would be the time to ask a few questions.

We're going to assume you've shared information regarding all of your prescription medications, vitamins and supplements, and herbal remedies. And we're trusting your caregiver is aware of any muscle problems you may have, or any family history of these. Lastly, you'll need to make sure your vitamin D level is normal, your thyroid gland is functioning properly, and your baseline liver studies are fine. All of these are important, not just for starting a statin, but also for your general health.

The first step will be to decide how strong a statin you need. Your physician will need to guide you with this one, but if your LDL is mildly elevated or your HDL is low but not dangerously so, one of the less potent agents might be appropriate. These would be pravastatin and fluvastatin. Remember, they cause fewer muscle problems, so this is a real consideration. On the other hand, should you have documented heart disease and really bad lipids, you and your doctor might need to reach for the big guns. Let's try to compare the strengths of these various medications.

One way to look at this is to compare the amount of drug it takes to lower one of your lipids by a specified percentage. Since LDL is the bad cholesterol and the one we really need to deal with, we'll use it in our example. And we'll use a reduction of 30 to 40 percent, since this would be a good starting point. For some people, this may be all they need to do.

To lower your LDL by 30 to 40 percent, you will need:

- rosuvastatin (Crestor)—5 mgs
- atorvastatin (Lipitor)—10 mgs
- simvastatin (Zocor)—20 mgs
- pravastatin (Pravachol)—40 mgs
- lovastatin (Mevacor)—40 mgs
- fluvastatin (Lescol)—80 mgs

This gives us an idea about relative strengths, and once again we see that pravastatin and fluvastatin are at the bottom of this list. But frequently this is not the determining factor in how we choose a statin. For most of my patients, and probably for you, the choice of a statin has to do with what your insurance company has to say and then ultimately about money.

You'll have to wait for another book from me to describe all the problems we face with our insurance companies and pharmaceutical plans. Suffice it to say that as a physician, I understand the dilemma and like many of my patients, I'm very frustrated. But today, drug cost is the major determinant in the accessibility of various medications. Let's see how these statins stack up in this regard.

This information comes from a current Internet database and I'm sure is subject to change. An individual's cost will vary, based on insurance plans, copays, choice of pharmacy, and even geographic location. Below are typical costs for a one-month supply of these drugs, along with their routine starting dose.

- Crestor (10 mgs)—$161
- Lipitor (10-20 mgs)—$130-178
- Simvastatin (20 mgs, generic)—$68
- Pravastatin (40 mgs, generic)—$46
- Lovastatin (10-20 mgs)—$12-16
- Fluvastatin (20 mgs)—$135

That's a wide range of costs, which underscores the point that money will be a factor in our choice. And if the time of day you take your medicine makes a difference to you, Crestor, Lipitor, and pravastatin can be taken at any time, while simvastatin, fluvastatin, and lovastatin should be taken at night or with your evening meal. The reasoning here—our bodies manufacture most of our cholesterol during the night, while we are fasting. Simvastatin, fluvastatin, and lovastatin are relatively short-acting drugs (about six hours) and will miss this window if taken too early during the day. The other statins are longer-acting, hence the flexibility in their dosing.

Lastly, many of our patients ask whether the "combination drugs" are appropriate for them to consider. Drug manufacturers have combined some interesting medicines, including the following:

Simvastatin + Ezetimibe
(a new class of cholesterol absorption inhibitor)
Lovastatin + niacin
Lipitor + amlodipine (a blood pressure medicine)
Simvastatin + niacin

While convenient, these are costly combinations, much more so than their individual components. As such, and because of the need to adjust the doses of the individual medicines, most experts don't typically recommend them. I have to agree.

So the choice of a statin is a bit complicated. As with most things, one size doesn't fit everyone, so talk with your physician and ask enough questions until you're comfortable with your decision.

34

What Are Some of the Other Drugs?

In addition to our statins, we have a couple of other options in our battle against elevated lipids. Let's take a look at these, when they should be used, potential benefits and side effects, and how much they cost.

We'll start with the *fibrates*. This group of medications includes gemfibrozil (Lopid) and fenofibrate (Tricor), and they are *fibric acid derivatives*. How these drugs work is not well understood, but it appears to be complicated and multifactored. They are effective in lowering triglyceride levels and that's where we use them most, though they do possess the ability to raise HDL levels as well. Their cost is in the range of $30/month for standard dosing.

There are some snags with these medicines. First, like the statins, fibrates can cause muscle problems. When they are added to a statin, the risk goes way up as well as the severity. More bothersome is current evidence that fibrates as a group may tend to increase all-cause mortality, increase noncardiac deaths, and have no effect on cardiovascular mortality. The risks are small but troubling. This will take more time to shake out, but it causes me to pause when I consider prescribing these drugs. This comes on the heels of one of the earlier drugs in this class, clofibrate, being associated with the development of several types of gastrointestinal cancers.

Another class of medications are the *bile acid sequestrants*. That's not a very enticing name, but it is descriptive. Cholesterol is constantly circulating throughout our bodies, mainly through our bloodstreams. But it also travels in a circuit that flows through our GI tracts. First it's absorbed in our intestines and is then taken up by our liver. There it is altered and attached to *bile salts,* which are secreted back into our intestines. Then they are absorbed again and taken back to our liver.

It makes sense that if you can block any part of this circuit, you might be able to interfere with the manufacture and metabolism of cholesterol. And that's just what these sequestrants accomplish. They sequester bile salts/cholesterol in our GI tracts by binding with them and blocking reabsorption. This lowers our blood levels of cholesterol as well as LDL. They're not as powerful as statins, but they can reduce these levels by anywhere from 10 to 25 percent, depending on the dose.

But in order to achieve these beneficial outcomes, we have to use relatively high doses of these drugs. As you would expect, this results in a significant incidence of side effects. Since they work in the GI tract (and are not absorbed themselves), this is where we have our problems, which include nausea, bloating, and cramping. Another potential side effect is the impact these drugs can have on some of the other medicines we might be taking. For instance, the absorption of Coumadin (a blood thinner), digoxin (a heart medicine) and fat-soluble vitamins (A, D, E, K) can be diminished, causing real problems.

What are some examples of bile acid sequestrants, and how much do they cost? Here's a list and what you can expect to pay for a month's treatment, based on a low to middle dosing.

- cholestyramine (Questran)—$30
- colestipol (Colestid)—$50
- colesevelam (Welchol)—$75

Colesevelam is interesting in that in addition to its lipid-lowering effects, it also appears to be able to help diabetics with their blood-sugar levels.

The real drawback with all of these drugs is their GI side effects. Many of our patients stop taking them because of that.

The last class of lipid-lowering agents we'll consider is currently represented by one drug—*ezetimibe* (Zetia). This is a new class of medication that inhibits the dietary absorption of cholesterol. It appears to be able to lower LDL levels by as much as 17 percent and can be used with a statin, possibly lowering the needed dosage of that drug. It's well-tolerated, with few side effects, and carries a price tag of about $60/month.

However, recent studies and experience with this medicine have turned up some problems. Its ability to lower the risk of heart disease has been challenged, and there is troubling evidence that it might in fact worsen plaque formation. We don't use much of it in our clinic at this time, and we'll see what happens with further research. If you're taking this medicine, talk with your doctor and see what they think.

To better help you grasp all this information about drug options, here's a quick overview of how these classes of drugs compare to our statin drugs regarding their ability to improve our lipids.

Drug Class	Lowers LDL	Raises HDL	Lowers Triglycerides
Statins	20-40%	5-10%	10-33%
Bile acid sequestrants	15-30%	0%	0%
Fibrates	10-15%	5-20%	35-50%
Niacin	10-25%	15-35%	25-30%
Ezetimibe	17%	1%	7-8%

From this chart we can see that statins have the greatest potential for lowering LDL levels, while niacin does the best job of raising HDL (we'll look closer at niacin in the next chapter). Finding the right medicine or combination is challenging, but it can be done. Questions remain as to whether we should be using the fibrates or ezetimibe. This area of our healthcare has exploded over the past few decades, and there's no reason to believe we won't have better, more effective medicines in the future—hopefully with fewer side effects and concerns.

35

Niacin

It was 8:30 a.m., and I sat in the kitchen in front of my computer, sorting through a long list of emails. Strange, my face felt hot—flushed. I was drinking coffee, thought that must be the reason, and scrolled through more messages.

Now my whole body felt flushed. I glanced at my forearms and saw…a lobster. I was beet-red, from head to toe. My skin was prickly, crawling, and drops of perspiration were forming on my forehead. This wasn't my coffee.

Many of you know what was going on here. I had decided to try some niacin in the hopes it would improve my borderline HDL. Taken with my morning handful of other supplements, I hadn't given it another thought. Not until I found myself peeling off my clothes and hurrying to a cold shower.

The flushing passed, as did my desire to take any more niacin. At least until recently. Let me tell you why.

Niacin (and its cousin nicotinic acid) is considered an *essential human nutrient.* Its deficiency can result in headaches, fatigue, skin and mouth lesions, anemia, and vomiting. Prolonged and significant deficiency can result in pellagra (a multisystem disease that we all learned about in medical school but which I've never seen).

For those interested in trivia, niacin is also known as vitamin B_3 because it was the third B vitamin to be identified. But it was also known as vitamin PP because of its "pellagra-preventive" properties. Hmm…maybe should have been PPP.

Naturally occurring niacin is found in a wide variety of foods, including chicken, fish, liver, avocados, nuts, dates, peanut butter, and even mushrooms. The daily requirements for this vitamin fall somewhere between 20 and 40 mgs/day. A reasonably healthy diet easily provides this amount.

Here we're interested in niacin because of its beneficial effects on our lipids. These were discovered in the mid-1950s, making this our oldest cholesterol/lipid lowering drug. So how does it work?

Niacin inhibits the formation of VLDL (see chapter 45), which ultimately results in a lower LDL level. It also raises our HDL level, something we know is protective of our heart and blood vessels. At adequate doses, that reduction can be as much as 30 to 35 percent, rivaling our statin drugs.

But what is an adequate dose? For individuals with elevated cholesterol and LDL levels associated with a normal or low HDL, it's probably going to take 1 to 2 grams of niacin/nicotinic acid a day. In order to achieve the maximal benefit in lowering LDL and VLDL levels, that dose might be as much as 3 grams/day. That's a lot more than the 40 mg average daily requirement.

How are we to get that much into our systems?

There are a couple of prescription formulations of niacin. Though more expensive than over-the-counter (OTC) products, they deliver a more dependable amount of active drug, and they generally cause less flushing. Dosing usually starts at 500 mgs/night for a month, and if well tolerated, can be increased 500 mgs each month until we reach our target of 1 to 2 grams/night.

It turns out there may be some problems with the myriad OTC products available to us. These are mainly due to the inconsistencies of active ingredients and to the fact that "nonflushing" varieties may be nonflushing for a good reason—they contain very little active niacin.

I was happy to learn I was in good company with my response to niacin. It seems that up to 80 percent of people who take this medication experience some degree of flushing. This is by far the most frequent side effect of the drug, and it can be very bothersome. The good news—the flushing usually lasts only a couple of weeks and then goes away. It can also be helped by making sure you are well-hydrated, take it at night, and take aspirin (325 mgs, not the 81 mg in a baby aspirin) or 200 mgs of ibu-profen thirty minutes before the niacin. Another trick is to take the medication with a snack or preferably a meal. The point is, the flushing will usually subside and can be helped by using these techniques.

Why go to all the trouble? If your lipids are out of line and for some reason you're unable to take a statin, niacin is the next batter up. It will be worth the effort to work through the flushing, should you experience it. Keep in mind that niacin by itself is an effective lipid-lowering drug. When taken with a statin, it can further lower total cholesterol and LDL levels, and help your HDL. At the same time, the combination can cause more side effects. Make sure you and your physician discuss this.

Aside from the flushing, what are the other potential side effects? There are a few, but they don't occur very often and usually at the higher end of dosing. We can see elevations in our liver enzymes, which if unrecognized, can cause hepatic damage. That's why it's important to frequently monitor these values when taking this or any other medication that can affect your liver.

We can also see elevations in blood sugar, making it important for those of us with diabetes to keep an eye on our glucose levels. Again, this doesn't happen very often. Nor does an increase in gout attacks in those with this disease, but it does happen, and is something we need to keep in mind.

When everything is considered, this is a safe and effective weapon in our fight against abnormal lipid levels. My advice is to work closely with your physician, stay away from any nonflushing OTC products, keep in mind the potential side effects, and work through any flushing problems, if you can.

I gave it another shot, tried the techniques listed here, and was able to take my niacin without any problems. Now the only time my face flushes is when someone reminds me of my alleged misbehavings in the ER.

36

Give Me the Details, Doc

Triglycerides

We've already talked a little about *triglycerides* and what these molecules look like. Just as a reminder, the basic building block here is a glycerol particle, to which are attached three (hence the *tri-*) fatty acids. These are simply chains of carbon atoms, much like the pop beads you might have played with as a child. The three chains are usually of varying lengths and of variable degrees of saturation, which has to do with the availability (or not) of open spaces for hydrogen atoms to attach. If all the spaces are filled, the fatty acid is said to be "saturated." If some are available, it's "unsaturated." This is important, as it affects the behavior of the molecule and whether or not it causes more harm than good.

When we talk about blood fats, we're almost always talking about the triglycerides floating around in our body. These are important factors in a lot of processes, and essential for our well-being. The best way to think about their role is as a transporter. They transport fat from the GI tract to the liver, and back and forth from the liver to adipose (fat) cells throughout our bodies.

Their main function is to serve as an energy source—both for storage (when we eat too much) and for fuel (when we need to burn something for energy). As a source of energy, triglycerides and their associated fatty acids are twice as efficient as carbohydrates. There are two sides to this sword.

When we need energy, our stores of fat provide a significant and efficient reservoir. But when we're trying to fit into last-year's-clothes and trying to lose some of that fat, it comes off very slowly and with a lot of effort. Yet we need this essential ability to store and preserve energy for a rainy day, when food isn't readily available.

That's some of the good news about triglycerides. Now for the bad. Most of us never experience that rainy day. We have too much to eat, much of it being unhealthy. Things start to go wrong when we have a lot of these triglycerides—fats—in our blood. And more than a third of Americans have elevated levels, putting a large number of us (one out of three) at risk for trouble. That may include you, so pay attention.

Hypertriglyceridemia, sometimes referred to as *hyperlipidemia*, has long been suspected of being associated with the development of heart disease. Over the past decade or so, mounting evidence indicates that this is in fact the case. Too much fat in your bloodstream is an *independent* risk factor for cardiovascular disease, meaning it can do this on its own, without an elevated cholesterol or LDL level. This makes sense, when you think about thick, milky fat floating through your major arteries.

We also know this is linked to the risk of certain kinds of strokes, particularly those caused by the sudden obstruction of the vessels that supply blood to critical areas of our brains.

And we learned earlier that elevated levels of blood fats can cause pancreatitis, an inflammatory condition of this important gland that can sometimes prove fatal.

So this is serious business, and something we need to know about. The diagnosis is made by simple blood studies. There aren't any symptoms to warn you of high levels, other than the infrequent appearance of yellowish, raised skin lesions (*xanthomas*), the serendipitous finding of an enlarged liver or spleen, or the infrequent but usually specific changes in the back of your eye (fatty deposits on our retinas).

But if our physician informs us that our triglyceride level is elevated, how did that happen? What causes this condition?

This comes about in two ways. The first is due to faulty metabolic regulation of the levels of our triglycerides and other fats. We either make too much, store too much, or don't break down and eliminate enough. These are almost always due to genetic disorders, and are inherited in a variety of ways. Not much to do here except make the correct diagnosis and manage the problem accordingly.

The other way is much more common. Fortunately, it usually lends itself to straightforward and effective treatments. This category is termed *acquired disorders*, of which there are many. They are *acquired*, meaning we are doing something to ourselves, or some condition, medication, or treatment is adversely affecting us. There are a bunch of these disorders, and we need to be aware of them.

- Obesity is a big factor here, with increasing BMIs causing lots of problems for us in lots of areas.

- Along with obesity, we now know that the ingestion of a high carbohydrate diet will elevate our triglycerides.

- Hypothyroidism (an underactive thyroid gland) is a common condition, and a well-known aggravator of our lipid status.

- Diabetes, especially in patients with poor blood-sugar control, is a significant factor.

- Renal failure and other kidney diseases have been implicated here.

- Blood fats are normally elevated during pregnancy, but can cause problems and may persist after delivery.

- Some forms of estrogen replacement can elevate lipid levels.

- Several medications have consistently been shown to elevate triglyceride levels. These include tamoxifen (an anticancer drug), the commonly used blood pressure medicines known as "beta blockers," and the frequently used "fluid pill," hydrochlorothiazide (HCTZ). Other medications will do this as well, including the often used anti-inflammatory drug prednisone.

- Recently, we have learned that many of the drugs in our expanding treatments for HIV will also significantly raise lipid levels.

That's a lot, and you might find yourself described somewhere in this list, or you might be aware of a family history of lipid problems. Whatever the cause, if our triglycerides are elevated, we need to know about it. The good news is that there are safe and effective ways to attack it.

37

The Buzz About Antioxidants

Who would have thought that oxygen could cause such a problem? We all know its role in a raging fire, right? Without oxygen the fire goes out, so something is going on here. In a way, the same thing is going on in our bodies. While we can't live without it, our friend O_2 can wreak havoc where we least expect it.

It turns out the oxygen molecule is highly reactive, meaning it can combine with other molecules to form what are called "reactive oxygen species"—free radicals. It's these free radicals that do the damage. Let's take a look at how this happens.

These radicals are themselves highly reactive and can cause chemical chain reactions. When these happen in a cell, significant damage can be done, even to the point of cell death. This is called *oxidative stress* and may be responsible for a lot of different disease processes. For instance, it may be a factor in the development of several cancers, as well as Parkinson's disease, Alzheimer's, rheumatoid arthritis, and in several of the complications we see with longstanding diabetes.

Here's an interesting and useful fact. In our cells, one of the reactive oxygen species that's produced is the familiar H_2O_2—hydrogen peroxide. It can start one of these chain reactions that may damage DNA, causing mutations and even cancer, and it can cause destruction of various proteins and enzymes.

Maybe interesting, but how is this useful? Hydrogen peroxide does the same thing to our tissues. We've all probably cleaned scrapes and cuts with this stuff and watched the bubbling, which we were told meant it was working. The bubbling was actually this very same oxidative reaction, and healthy tissue was being damaged. Remember it turning white? We now know this treatment should be avoided, and these scrapes and cuts cleaned with simple soap and water. *That* should be useful.

Regarding our lipids, we know that the oxidation of LDL molecules appears to trigger the process of plaque formation in our arteries, leading to various cardiovascular diseases. We also know that the more LDL we have floating around, the greater the potential for this to occur. We need to keep in mind that this oxidation process is normal and goes on all the time in our bodies. If you remember your high school chemistry classes, it's that old oxidation-reduction reaction—different molecules passing hydrogen atoms back and forth.

But enough chemistry. How does this affect our health?

This is where the *antioxidants* come into play. It's all about balance— too much oxidation going on and we have oxidative stress. Not enough, and things don't get done in our cells. If you had to choose, you should try to avoid the stress thing. This causes damage, and here we find one more example of how our bodies have been "fearfully and wonderfully made" to make sure this damage doesn't happen. Several molecules circulate throughout our bodies "scavenging" these free radicals—reacting with them and neutralizing them. These are our naturally occurring antioxidants. The key is to make sure we have enough of these on board.

These beneficial actions of antioxidants have stimulated a lot of interest in the medical community. If we can increase the amounts of antioxidants in our bodies, we should be able to reduce the incidence of some of the disease processes we just discussed.

At first, a lot of the studies were observational and not carefully done. The findings were positive, and there was a lot of noise regarding the benefits of several readily available supplements. These predominately included vitamins A (beta-carotene), C, and E. For a while, antioxidants were all the rage, with exuberant and unsubstantiated health claims appearing in the media almost weekly. This led to a more measured, thorough investigation of these supplements in order to determine how they might best be used—or whether they should even be used in the first place.

We now have a lot of solid information, coming from large and multiple randomized studies. Unfortunately, dietary supplementation with vitamins A, C, and E doesn't confer any significant benefit for combatting a multitude of diseases. These include the neurological diseases we discussed, as well as several types of cancer and cardiovascular diseases. Disappointing, since this would be a simple and inexpensive way to impact these devastating conditions.

There is a silver lining, though. What we *have* demonstrated is that these diseases can be positively impacted by a diet high in fruits and vegetables—particularly those high in antioxidants. Why these foods work while the supplements don't remains a mystery. It may have something to do with the way these foods are digested and metabolized, or it may be the presence of something as yet undiscovered. Whatever the reason, the consumption of foods rich in antioxidants should be part of our daily diets.

Just what are these fruits and vegetables? And where else can we find these antioxidants? Here's a partial list of foods and beverages that contain a lot of antioxidants and are easily found. In descending order of their antioxidant levels (according to some researchers):

- coffee (yes, that's right)
- tea (a multitude of varieties)
- red wine
- blueberries
- walnuts
- oranges
- cinnamon (we're going to look at spices later)
- broccoli

This is not an exhaustive list, but there should be something here for everyone. And the good news is that you don't have to consume mountains of these to experience a significant benefit to your health.

38

You Can Change Your Jeans But Not Your Genes

It's tough enough trying to change your lifestyle in order to get your lipids in order. But when your own genetic code is working against you, it's doubly—maybe triply—difficult.

Lipid disorders are frequently caused by one or more genetic abnormalities—gene mutations at various sites. They can involve cholesterol itself, triglycerides, HDL, or LDL. Since it's the LDL that causes most of our problems, that's where our focus will be in this chapter.

These disorders result in either too much LDL being produced, not enough being removed from our bodies, or a combination of each. A growing number of these conditions are being discovered and defined, making it difficult to keep up with this expanding area of our medical knowledge. Fortunately, two of these disorders seem to cause a majority of the problems we see in our day-to-day practice—familial hypercholesterolemia (FH) and familial combined hyperlipidemia (FCHL).

We're going to refer to these inherited disturbances of our LDL metabolism as *familial* ("characteristic of a family") since that's how these cases are usually discovered. Clusters of family members will develop premature heart disease (defined as occurring earlier than fifty-five years of age in men and sixty-five years in women), sometimes at a very early age (as young as twenty to thirty years). Not everyone in the family will develop heart disease, though they have the genetic predisposition. This is encouraging, and has led many researchers to the conclusion that the manifestation of this disorder is strongly influenced by such factors as diet (low saturated-fat intake) and low rates of obesity. Environment *does* influence heredity.

Not everyone is so lucky. Some genetic disorders will manifest themselves regardless of lifestyle, and this happens at an early age. That's the reason we need to be aware of this, make the diagnosis as soon as we can, and start treating it.

Before we look at diagnosing these disorders, let's consider the inheritance patterns. This is fairly straightforward, so bear with me.

FH is a *dominantly* inherited condition, meaning it will be manifested if one gene in the pair is mutated and one is normal. The bad gene dominates the good one. In this scenario, each child has a 50-50 chance of inheriting the mutated gene. The risk of early coronary disease depends on the gender of the child and looks like this:

- Of the males with the mutated gene, 50 percent will develop heart disease by the age of fifty.

- All of the affected males will develop it by age seventy.

- Make sure you're sitting down for this one, because it's really scary. Of affected male children, 85 percent will have a heart attack before the age of sixty.

- Females fare a little better, with 15 percent developing heart disease before fifty and 75 percent by the age of seventy.

This is serious business, so we need to identify these individuals and do what we can to lessen the impact of this disorder.

Now for the identification part. First, we should be able to see a problem with family history. That's why this piece of information is so important. Next, we want to know about heart attacks at an early age and whether one or both parents had problems with their LDL levels—especially if they were resistant to most commonly used treatments. Many of us won't know the answers to that, but as time passes, more of this information will be available to family members.

The physical exam might also be important, with evidence of cholesterol deposits on the elbows and knees (tendon xanthomas) and the cholesterol deposits on the eyelids that we've previously discussed (xanthelasmas).

That should lead us to checking blood work and finding elevated levels of cholesterol and LDL, clinching the diagnosis.

Now about treatment. As we said, this is serious business and needs to be addressed as early as possible. The management will follow the outline we've looked at before, with special attention paid to any needed lifestyle changes: diet, exercise, weight loss, and no smoking. We haven't talked a lot about the dangers of cigarettes, but they are killers and their elimination is critical.

Lipid-lowering medications are usually effective, but may require higher dosing to achieve the typically recommended aggressive goals. And supplements such as fish oil and niacin will probably be utilized as well. We need to pull out all the guns—large and small.

This is complex and confusing stuff. The take-home message is to be aware of the genetic component of lipid abnormalities, make sure you know as much about your family's health history as possible, and if you fall into this category, don't give up hope. With the help of your physician and your own dedication and commitment, this can be managed.

39

You Gotta Know Your Numbers

Procrastination

Freddie Jacobs rested a huge, heavy hand on my shoulder. I turned and had to look up into the eyes of the six-foot-six general surgeon.

"Well, Robert, looks like you were right about that Alexander boy. His appendix was just about five minutes from poppin'. But he's going to do fine and should be headed home in the morning." He glanced around the department, then studied the patient ID board. "Doesn't look like you've got any business for me up there."

"We're okay for now. But the night's young."

Freddie chuckled, his barrel chest resonating beside me. "Just call if you need anything."

He headed out the ambulance entrance, and I walked to the medicine room to grab some supplies. The window in the room opened onto the ER parking lot, and I watched as Freddie lumbered up the gently sloping hill toward his car. He stopped, reached into his lab coat, and took out a pack of cigarettes. I cringed a little as he lit one and took a deep drag, blowing a huge cloud of smoke over his head as he ambled on. He knew better, but some habits don't die until you do.

I was about to turn away when Freddie stopped again, reached down, and began rubbing his right calf. It was one of those things you notice but don't think about, and then file away.

A few days later, Freddie Jacobs did the same thing, and this time I paid attention. He was walking down the hallway in the ER and stopped just before reaching the nursing station. He scowled, leaned over, and began rubbing that same calf. He straightened, shook his head, and walked over to where I stood.

"Freddie, what's going on with that leg?" I said.

"Just some cramps I've been getting. Mainly that right leg, but starting to feel some pain on the left side too. I think I must be overdoing my exercise program. My wife bought a stationary bike, and I've been trying to put in fifteen or twenty minutes at least three times a week."

"When did you start that?" I was having difficulty not smiling. The image of this huge man pedaling away on a small bike, probably smoking a cigarette, would be highly entertaining.

"Almost a week now." He grinned at me. "But don't you worry. I'm going to keep at it until I lose some weight and get in shape."

"And those cigarettes?"

He patted his lab-coat pocket and shook his head. "That's going to take awhile. I know I need to stop, but one thing at a time."

We were caught up with our patients, and I motioned to the empty stretcher of room 3.

"Come on over here and let me look at those legs. When's the last time you had your blood pressure checked or any kind of examination?" Doctors are indeed the worst patients.

"Been awhile, but don't trouble yourself. I'm fine."

I was already in the room and stood by the stretcher, motioning for him to join me.

Muttering something I couldn't understand, he rambled into the room and plopped down heavily on the bed.

Lori Davidson, the charge nurse this morning, followed us into the room and took his blood pressure.

"One sixty over one hundred." Lori frowned at the affable surgeon.

"Might be a little nervous or something," Freddie mumbled.

I rolled up the pant legs of his surgical scrubs and searched for a pulse in his right ankle. Nothing. My fingers continued to probe and prod his foot, noting its coolness and lack of hair. There was no hair on his lower legs as well, a sign of poor blood flow.

I was frowning.

"What's the matter, Robert?"

"We've got a problem here, Freddie."

We had *big* problems. In addition to his elevated blood pressure, cigarette smoking, and poor blood flow in his legs, Freddie's blood work revealed a markedly elevated cholesterol. His LDL was twice normal.

I convinced him to cancel his afternoon office appointments, and we got some vascular studies of his legs. Not surprisingly, we found his main arteries to be almost completely obstructed, narrowed by massive deposits of cholesterol. That would explain the pain in his legs—not enough blood flow to his muscles when he did much of any walking. It's the same problem that causes angina—narrowed blood vessels can't provide enough oxygen to a person's heart muscle. I knew we would soon be looking there as well.

"Freddie, how long has this been going on?"

He sighed and shook his head. "A couple of months, maybe more. I've just been too busy to do anything about it."

Freddie had known. He had seen too many legs just like his own and had amputated many of them himself.

I understood his anxiety, and his fear. It was my turn to lay a hand on *his* shoulder.

"We need to have you looked at—right now."

40

Complementary and Alternative Medicine

We're frequently asked about alternative treatments for many common ailments—especially what we think about their effectiveness. It all depends, but first let's define these terms.

Complementary medicine refers to using a nonmainstream approach *along with* mainstream medicine. *Alternative medicine* refers to the use of a nonmainstream approach *in place of* conventional, mainstream medicine.

A true alternative approach to a medical problem—for instance, treating bacterial pneumonia with poultices—is not very common. It's much more likely we'll combine nonmainstream and conventional treatments if we're convinced of the effectiveness of both.

For our discussion here, we'll use the acronym CAM, which stands for "complementary and alternative medicine." It encompasses all the various nonmainstream treatments available to us. The margins begin to blur a little with the passage of time. What was earlier considered to be CAM has become more conventional. A few examples are the utilization of fish oil in the treatment of elevated triglyceride levels and niacin to elevate low HDL levels. Prior to that would be the native Peruvians' discovery of the medicinal use of the bark of the cinchona tree. It found widespread use as a treatment for malaria (quinine) and a cardiac medicine (quinidine), variations of which are still in use today.

How common is the use of CAM therapies in the United States? It appears that one in five of us will employ some form of this treatment, with the choices including acupuncture, ayurveda (a system of Hindu traditional medicine), homeopathy, Chinese or Oriental medicine, chiropractic, massage, body movement therapies, tai chi, yoga, dietary supplements, herbal medicine, biofeedback, electromagnetic therapy, qigong (balancing your chi or "life energy"), meditation, hypnosis, and even art, dance, and music. Whew.

In the US, the most frequently used CAM therapies (in descending order) are: herbal remedies, breathing meditation, other forms of meditation, chiropractic manipulation, yoga, diet-based therapy, progressive relaxation, and megavitamin therapy. Interestingly, the British National Health Service lists their three most commonly employed CAM therapies as acupuncture, aromatherapy, and chiropractic. I wonder if that's a spinal manipulation with a needle in your ear and a rose in your nose.

The problem we face with CAM therapies is determining their effectiveness and safety. We have the same dilemma with our conventional treatments, whether they be pharmaceutical, surgical, or other (such as radiation therapy). It all comes down to performing rigorous and reproducible research. That takes money, and frequently a lot of it. Our pharmaceutical companies have it to spend, and they fund much (many think *too* much) of our ongoing medical research. They need to prove their latest medicines will work and are safe so they can get them to the market.

As you can imagine, there's probably not a lot of research going on with ayurveda or regarding the use of dance for depression. When it does happen, most studies fail to demonstrate any beneficial outcomes with many CAM therapies. There have been a couple of noteworthy exceptions. The practice of tai chi has been shown to significantly reduce the incidence of falls among our elderly, probably due to better conditioning and balance. And several types of acupuncture have proven effective for selected conditions, including low-back pain and migraine headaches. Probably not better than conventional treatments and usually more expensive, but it seems to work. With the passage of time, many of these CAM therapies, or elements of them, may merge into the conventional.

Until then, I'm going to keep an open mind but rely on reputable journal reports and the results of well-designed and large studies. If you're considering a CAM therapy, talk with your physician. If he or she tries to discourage you and you forge ahead anyway, just be sure to let him or her know.

After all, that next tree you chew on may be the secret to everlasting youth, or at least a cure for baldness.

41

Green Tea and Red Yeast Rice

Sounds like #47 at your favorite Chinese restaurant. Actually green tea *is* one of our favorite alternative medications, easily falling into the top ten in total annual sales. Red rice—not so much, but still bought and consumed by millions of Americans. What do we know about these products, and what good do they do?

Green tea has been around for thousands of years, with its earliest history tracing back to China. Even way back then, its purported health benefits were many and varied. Here are some of the claims:

- Acts as a stimulant, improving brain function (thought to be due to its caffeine)
- Contains several active *antioxidants* (polyphenols)
- Increases fat burning and boosts your metabolic rate (Remember, these are *claims*.)
- May lower the risk of developing certain types of cancer
- Reduces the incidence of Alzheimer's
- May help you live longer, especially if your drink four to five cups a day
- Can lower your risk of developing type 2 diabetes
- May reduce your risk of cardiovascular disease

This final point is the one we're interested in, since many of the other claims are not grounded in solid evidence. Here's what we know about the effects of green tea on our lipids, and how these effects could be beneficial for our hearts and vascular systems.

Some studies have demonstrated a reduction in LDL and total cholesterol in individuals who regularly consume green tea. While consistently present, these changes in lipids are small—only a few percentage points. Interestingly, these same studies showed a reduction in blood pressure, both systolic and diastolic (the upper and lower numbers). Again, these were small changes. There is no evidence of consistent improvements in HDL levels.

Additionally, in the studies comparing green and black tea, while the findings for green tea remained constant and reproducible, those for black tea were not. Some research demonstrates positive effects for black tea; other investigations reveal none.

One important point here is that the consumption of green or black teas did not produce any negative side effects or health problems. Tea has been around for quite a while, and some lurking danger would have reared its head long ago.

The bottom line: drinking green tea is probably a good idea. Two or three cups a day might help your lipids—maybe even your blood pressure. If you prefer to take a capsule (which is what I do), be aware of the usual cautions with alternative supplements—the actual amounts of active ingredients vary from product to product. Check the label, keeping in mind the information presented might not be completely accurate.

Now let's consider *red yeast rice*. This is interesting stuff and representative of a lot of the benefits and problems with "complementary and alternative medications." It's also been around for hundreds—maybe thousands—of years, principally used in Chinese cuisine and medicine. It's a *fermented* product, hence the "yeast" in its name.

As with green tea, multiple health claims surround red yeast rice. These include the following:

- Lowers cholesterol levels (We'll be talking about this one.)

- Helps soothe indigestion, diarrhea, and an upset stomach

- Enhances circulation—apparently the primary reason for its inclusion in Chinese medicine
- Helps those with diabetes (Again, these are claims.)
- Can reduce pain when combined with several other herbs

But what do we really know here? Probably the most important fact is that red yeast rice contains substances called *monacolins*—chemicals that act like our statin drugs. It turns out that one of these monacolins is the active ingredient in the statin drug lovastatin. That explains red yeast rice's ability to lower cholesterol levels. And it can do just that—daily consumption of red yeast rice can lower both total cholesterol and LDL.

The amounts of monacolins in different red yeast rice products vary, providing anywhere from 2 to 5 mgs of the active drug each day. That compares to the usual daily doses of 20 to 40 mgs found in prescription lovastatin. And you can get the same muscle aches and pains with red yeast rice that we experience with the FDA-approved variety. Since 2 to 5 mgs is a small amount of lovastatin, something else must be present in red yeast rice to account for this—we just don't know yet what it is.

What we *do* know is that red yeast rice products contain variable levels of lovastatin, which can prove dangerous to many of us, especially those with liver problems. This is what led the FDA to try to ban sales of red yeast rice in this country—without success. Manufacturers have found ways to circumvent these regulations, and their products are still readily available—and still potentially harmful. You just don't know what you're getting.

And there's another problem. An investigation of multiple red yeast rice products found that several contained a chemical called *citrinin*—a substance known to cause serious kidney damage. Again, you just don't know what you're getting.

The bottom line with red yeast rice? There's no evidence that it helps individuals with diabetes or that it improves your circulation. We do know it can improve your lipids, but at a potentially serious price. This is something you need to avoid.

One further cautionary note: If you're taking this supplement, let your physician know. It's that important.

42

No More!
Vitamin A

It wasn't very long ago that vitamin A was one of the darlings of the preventive medicine gurus and one of the bestselling supplements at health food stores. It was touted as a powerful antioxidant, which it is. As such, it should prove useful in our fight against the cardiovascular disease epidemic in this country. That didn't pan out so much, largely because of what we've learned about this essential nutrient. Let's start at the beginning.

Vitamins are substances that can't be made in our bodies and must be ingested. Without them, we get into trouble, and there are well-defined deficiency conditions. Fortunately, we need only a small amount of these for proper metabolic functioning and good health.

Vitamin A was the first of these to be discovered—hence the *A*. Next were the B vitamins, then the...well, you get the idea. The early Egyptians knew about this substance, though they didn't know what to call it. They observed that night blindness (a condition caused by a lack of vitamin A) could be cured by feeding the patient liver, an excellent source of this supplement.

As we began to learn more about various vitamins, we discovered there were two types—the fat-soluble variety and the water-soluble ones. This turned out to be important, since this chemistry affects their availability in the body as well as their toxicity at high levels. The water-soluble vitamins (the B complex, C, and others) do just that—they dissolve in water.

They move freely through our bodies and are readily excreted through our kidneys and urine. It's hard to overdose on these.

On the other hand, the fat-soluble vitamins (A, D, and E) are readily absorbed by our fatty tissue and can accumulate there, sometimes to dangerous levels. That's why we need only small amounts of these. And it's why they accumulate in specific organs in our body such as the liver (80 to 85 percent stored here) and skin (yes the skin *is* an organ). This point is important with regards to their toxicity, which we'll discuss in a moment.

What is a little different and confusing about vitamin A is that it exists in two forms. The first is beta-carotene, a water-soluble particle that is converted to the fat-soluble active form of the vitamin known as retinol or retinoic acid. (Sound a little familiar? A form of retinol A is used topically for the treatment of acne.)

Beta-carotene is found in green leafy vegetables as well as in carrots and sweet potatoes. Retinol usually comes from an animal source such as egg yolk, butter, liver, and kidney. (Who eats kidneys?)

As with many vitamins, minerals, and other substances, we have learned much about them from what happens when they are deficient in our bodies. What does their lack in our bodies cause? With vitamin-A deficiency, the problems usually relate to visual issues: night blindness and sometimes complete blindness, as well as problems with bone development and growth.

Since a reasonably healthy diet contains more than enough vitamin A for our needs, we seldom see this deficiency in the United States. However, in parts of the world where an adequate diet is often missing, as many as half a million children become blind each year, and many of them die. This problem has been the target of several organizations where the distribution of this simple and inexpensive vitamin can easily prevent these problems and make a difference in the lives of many.

What about the toxicity of vitamin A? This is interesting as well. Water-soluble beta-carotene seldom if ever causes any problems—passing quickly through our systems and being eliminated. It's the fat-soluble retinol that's the culprit.

There are two types of poisoning here—acute and chronic. *Acute vitamin-A toxicity* occurs when a massive amount is ingested, usually over 600,000 internal units (IU). To put that in perspective, our recommended daily allowance (RDA) is about 2,000 to 3,000 IU. Acute toxicity can happen with an intentional overdose, but normally it's due to an unintentional poisoning. As a tragic example, while exploring parts of the Arctic in the 1500s, several European scientists became sick and some died after eating the livers of polar bears. Their symptoms were classic for acute toxicity: nausea, vomiting, blurred vision, incoordination, seizures, and sometimes death.

Chronic vitamin-A poisoning is more common, and by definition occurs over time, usually in regular amounts more than ten times our RDA—25,000 to 30,000 IU. Interestingly, this amount has been found in many over-the-counter supplements. The symptoms of chronic toxicity include hair loss, bone and muscle pain, visual problems, incoordination, and liver damage.

You might be familiar with a common and benign manifestation of vitamin-A "overdose." Infants and toddlers who are fed a lot of carrot-based baby food and pureed green leafy vegetables can sometimes develop a yellowish tinge to their skin. Remember this vitamin is stored in the skin, and the condition is called *carotenemia*. It can be confused with jaundice, a more serious problem, but the yellow skin quickly clears when the intake of these foods is reduced.

Let's get back to the significant antioxidant qualities of this vitamin. When researchers became aware of this, it was logical to investigate it is as a possible preventive intervention for cardiovascular disease. This is another instance where we got the cart before the horse. Vitamin-A supplements (retinol, the active and fat-soluble kind) were readily available and frequently recommended as something we should all be taking.

However, once high-quality studies were conducted, several troubling issues emerged. Vitamin A and its precursor, beta-carotene, did not show any benefits for our cardiovascular health. Worse yet, there was evidence that its supplementation may be associated with a *worsening* of heart disease and an increase in the incidence of lung and colon cancer. It was time to put a *whoa!* on that horse, and that's what happened.

Supplementation with vitamin A or beta-carotene should absolutely be avoided, unless you have an established deficiency. Should a friend, relative, or your healthcare provider recommend this, gently decline and offer them a carrot.

43

Probably No More:
Vitamin E

Vitamin E is another of our fat-soluble vitamins. It has an interesting history, beginning in the early years of the last century.

Apparently two researchers were studying the effects of various diets on rats and discovered that one group unexpectedly developed infertility. They added an extract of several grains to their diet and quickly corrected the problem. Not knowing what had actually been the active agent, they simply termed it the "anti-sterility factor." A few years later, vitamin E, the fifth vitamin, was identified. Since it had cured the problem of infertility among these lab animals, the active ingredient was named *toco-pherol* from the Greek *toc* (child) and *pherol* (to bring forth). And we still refer to the active component of vitamin E as alpha-tocopherol. So there's your medical history lesson for today.

We now know that vitamin E is one of the *essential* nutrients for humans (remember, that means we aren't able to manufacture it ourselves) and does several important things for us. It is a potent antioxidant, and as such protects our cell membranes—including those of red blood cells—from oxidation and premature destruction. It also acts as a free radical scavenger, tracking down these harmful molecules and neutralizing them. We discussed earlier these radicals and the damage they are thought to inflict in various parts of our bodies.

One of the harmful actions of these particles has to do with the triggering and initiation of cancer cells—carcinogenesis. Another role involves the process of atherosclerosis and plaque formation in our arteries. In this chapter we're mainly concerned with that plaque business and how we can keep it from happening.

Once again, a lot of what we know about vitamin E comes from our experience when its levels are low. Some of these disorders are manifested by incoordination and gait disturbances, while others have to do with fertility (remember those lab rats). As we would expect, vitamin E deficiency can cause red blood-cell membranes to be easily damaged by free radicals (oxidants) with a resultant anemia. This can be especially serious in a newborn.

Fortunately, most American diets contain more than adequate amounts of this nutrient from meat, eggs, various oils, and leafy vegetables, and we seldom see these problems. They are usually associated with diseases with decreased fat absorption (liver damage, pancreatic insufficiency, and Crohn's disease) and are accompanied by deficiencies in the other fat-soluble vitamins.

As far as what goes on in our arteries, we know that LDL (the bad cholesterol) forms part of the plaques that almost all of us have. When that LDL is oxidized, it starts a process that damages the underlying lining of our vessels, which causes specific cells to migrate to the plaque and try to cool things off. The plaque grows, more damage is done, and we have a bigger problem. What we want is less LDL floating around in the first place, and we want antioxidants readily available to make sure whatever LDL we have in our vessel walls remains calm. Vitamin E is one of those antioxidants.

Theoretically, high levels of this vitamin should protect our blood vessels. So far, no compelling evidence supports this. The same is true for any benefit of vitamin E supplementation with the prevention of cancer, stroke, liver disease, and dementia. Studies are ongoing, but the jury is still out.

Yet many of us are taking this supplement, sometimes encouraged to do so by our healthcare provider. If there's no solid proof for it helping us, what's the potential downside? Can too much of it be harmful?

Let's start with the recommended daily allowance for a healthy adult. This is going to be 15 mg—the equivalent of 22 international units (IU), and a little less for children. Compare that with most health-food supplements, which contain anywhere from 50 to 400 IU. The "tolerable upper intake level" (UL) is thought to be around 1,500 IU in adults, though some experts think this number is too high. They have reported symptoms of toxicity with amounts far below that UL. Remember, these are the amounts we get with supplements in addition to dietary vitamin E.

But what problems are we going to experience with too much of this vitamin? A couple of these are very troubling. The most bothersome is that some evidence suggests supplementation of more than 400 IU a day is associated with an increased risk of "all-cause mortality"—meaning too much raises your chances of dying from just about everything. That doesn't give me a very warm and fuzzy feeling.

More commonly, toxicity manifests itself with bleeding issues. Alpha-tocopherol—the active ingredient—interferes with our normal clotting mechanisms, and there is an increased risk of stroke and major bleeding problems. Again, not very warm and fuzzy.

Several years ago, I decided to add vitamin E to my supplement regimen—400 IU a day. This was before I learned of the all-cause-mortality research. At some point I came across some information that higher levels of vitamin E might be even *better* for you. I found some 800 IU capsules and gave that a try. Less than a week later, I got out of the shower one morning, looked in the mirror, and discovered a large subconjunctival hemorrhage in my right eye. Actually, this is not *in* the eye but just under the conjunctiva and overlying the white part. Pretty scary when it happens, but not really serious unless it's caused by a significant underlying disease. Many of us have these, occurring spontaneously after sneezing, bearing down, or lifting a piano.

I had never had one, and immediately ran through the list of the worst possibilities. Then I remembered the vitamin E and the big dose I was taking. A quick review of the literature and a phone call to my ophthalmologist confirmed that the tocopherol was the culprit. He had seen quite a few individuals who developed these hemorrhages after taking vitamin E—especially if they were also taking low-dose aspirin every day (which would be me).

"Robert, why in the world are you taking that much vitamin E?"

"John, you're breaking up," I said, and quickly ended the call.

So where are we? I stopped taking any vitamin E years ago. There's no convincing evidence that it does any good, and I've seen the potential harm it can cause. At present, this is one of those supplements that should be avoided. There's a chance that further evidence will demonstrate a definite role for this vitamin in the prevention of heart disease, or cancer, or dementia—but we don't have it yet. For now, save your money.

44

Things You Need to Avoid

As we have seen, a lot of people are taking a lot of herbal medicines and over-the-counter supplements. We've talked about some of the safety issues with these alternative treatments, but this is serious business and we need to examine it more closely.

We're dealing with different kinds of medical problems here, some that involve the supplement or herb itself, some may be herb-herb interactions, while others are prescription drug-herb complications.

Let's start with medical problems caused by the supplement or herb itself.

As a historical reminder, *ephedra* (also known as *ma huang*) was imported into this country and promoted for weight loss and athletic enhancement. It didn't take very long for problems to surface following its use. Hypertension, heart attacks, strokes, seizures, deaths. The FDA banned its use and it has disappeared from this country, but not before causing a lot of damage and grief. Most of the other substances we'll be considering are still readily available, so we need to know about them.

In earlier chapters we discussed the problems with vitamins A and E. The bottom line was that no one needs to be taking A or beta-carotene, and few of us should be taking vitamin E. Vitamin E can be helpful if a deficiency is likely, but the dose shouldn't exceed 400 international units (IU) a day.

Several herbal products have been found to contain dangerous contaminants, including heavy metals. *Saint-John's-wort* is one of these, with lead being the offending agent. The difficulty continues to be quality assurance with its manufacture and the purity of its ingredients. This proves true for all herbal medicines.

The blossoms of *germander* have been used for various liver ailments. Ironically, this herb itself can cause nausea, vomiting, jaundice, and liver failure.

Chaparral is a plant found in the southwestern United States and is related to the creosote bush. That sounds tasty. It's been used for hundreds of years as an antibacterial and antifungal medication. It's also been touted to help with diarrhea, upper respiratory-tract infections, chronic skin conditions, and even rheumatism (whatever that is). It can cause an acute hepatitis, with significant elevations of liver enzymes, bilirubin, and ultimately jaundice.

Pennyroyal is used to flavor herbal teas and is purported to aid with digestive problems, liver disorders, gout, colds, and skin diseases. Acute toxicity manifests as GI distress, confusion, and seizures. It doesn't take much of this oil to cause problems, with only one tablespoon potentially resulting in death.

Who would think *mistletoe* would be listed here. Aside from its ability to induce kissing, it has been claimed to be an effective treatment for hypertension, dizziness, joint pain, seizures, and asthma. Impressive, but it can also induce hepatitis. Whether this is due to mistletoe itself or to some contaminant is unknown. Another example of not knowing what you're getting.

Kava kava has been used for centuries, with claims of relieving anxiety, menstrual cramps, and insomnia. Its use can lead to liver injury, liver failure, and even death. The exact mechanism of how this happens isn't known, but the dangers of this herb outweigh its potential usefulness.

Black cohosh and *green tea extracts* are extensively utilized in this country, and some studies support their usefulness—green tea with weight loss and black cohosh with menopausal symptoms. Some reports of liver injury with these herbs should cause us to be cautious with their use. This happens rarely, and as always, we need to balance the potential benefit with the possible harm.

We mentioned possible *herb-herb interactions*. There are a multitude of possibilities here, the diagnosis of which is compounded by several factors. The first is that most of us don't tell our healthcare providers about the alternative medications we are using. They don't show up on the radar and don't enter into any consideration of what might be causing a problem. The second factor with these products is the possibility of contamination, impurities, and unreliable dosage amounts. This makes medical problems associated with herb-herb interactions difficult to assess.

Regarding *herb-drug interactions*, here are a couple of well-documented and problematic examples.

Ginkgo biloba, purported but never proved to improve memory or help with Alzheimer's, has significant antiplatelet properties and can interfere with our clotting mechanisms. For a person taking Coumadin, NSAIDS, aspirin, or other blood thinners, this can prove disastrous. It's tough enough managing a patient taking Coumadin without throwing another blood thinner into the mix. If you insist on taking this herb, please let your physician know. The combination with other medicines can be deadly.

The normal metabolism of Saint-John's-wort is very similar to that of other important medications. When the wort is in your system, it can impact the effectiveness of various drugs, including cyclosporine (resulting in transplant rejection), oral contraceptives (another mouth to feed), Coumadin again (bleeding), and antiretroviral therapy for HIV infections (treatment failure). Once more, you have to balance the gain with the pain.

As you can see, a lot of these problems involve the liver. That's where our treatment of lipid disorders gets involved. Individuals taking statin drugs may develop liver toxicity if their medication is combined with some of these herbal products. As we noted earlier, this is serious business.

That's a lot of information. Just be careful if you're considering adding an herbal supplement to your diet. Problems abound, and the upside for most of these remains very cloudy. If you're interested in more information, here are some helpful resources.

- Natural Medicines Comprehensive Database (www.natural database.com)
- Consumer Lab (www.consumerlab.com)
- National Institutes of Health National Center for Complementary and Alternative Medicine, "Herbs at a Glance" fact sheets (nccam.nih.gov/health/herbsataglance.htm)

—⩗⊶⩗⊶⩗⊶⩗⊶⩗⊶⩗⊶⩗—

45

Give Me the Details, Doc

The Other Stuff

We need to know about a couple of other things, one of which is found on our lipid lab report—the VLDL.

This is the **Very Low Density** Lipoprotein, another of our "carrier" molecules. Its major components are triglycerides (the major transporter of these fats) and a specific type of lipoprotein—apolipoprotein C-III. When its levels in our blood are normal, it performs its function of storing and eliminating the lipids it's carrying. But when the level of VLDL is high, we have an increased risk of atherosclerotic cardiovascular disease. This is felt to be due in part to the bad effects of too much triglyceride, but also to the actions of the apolipoprotein C-III itself.

This is another of those bad actors, and it exerts its harmful effects by causing inflammation in our blood-vessel walls (and we know where that leads). At high levels, it also prevents the needed breakdown of some of our other fats, including triglycerides. This leads to another set of problems. And finally, this molecule has the ability to interfere with the work of a chemical that maintains a healthy endothelial cell (the cells that line the inside of our arteries).

While this lab value is listed on most if not all lipid reports, most healthcare providers don't address it because they're not exactly sure what to do with it. That's going to change as we learn more about how all these lipids and carriers and macrophages (those good scavenger cells) interact.

The next thing we need to know about is *not* reported on that lab slip—the *chylomicron*—and it turns out to be one of the major lipoproteins in our blood. In medical lingo, *chyle*, which stems from the Greek root meaning "the juice of plants or animals," refers to the thin, creamy liquid that circulates in our lymph system. These chylomicrons are very large particles that carry dietary lipids. These are the fats that are rapidly absorbed from your GI tract after you eat a cheeseburger, a rack of bacon, or a can of Spam. (For those of you younger than forty, this isn't a reference to your email screening function.) The more fat we eat, the more that is absorbed, and the more that needs to be carried first to our liver and eliminated or deposited in our adipose tissue.

A certain amount of chylomicrons are necessary to handle our dietary intake, but when they become elevated and stay that way, they become components of the foam cells that we know lead to plaque formation.

An interesting condition called *chylomicronemia* refers to a persistently elevated level of chylomicrons, even after a person fasts for twelve hours and isn't dumping more fat into their stomach and intestines. This is one of the genetic conditions that affects many of us, and it might have been what afflicted Clyde Anderson back in chapter 3. It's manifested by a thick, creamy plasma due to the abundance of chylomicrons, VLDL, and triglycerides. While the appearance of our blood serum might be alarming, the real danger comes in the form of a significant increase in our risk for heart disease.

Additionally, this disorder can lead to memory loss, abdominal pain, pancreatitis, and those skin lesions we discussed earlier—xanthomas. Again, this is not usually reported with our routine lipids, but an observant lab tech will notice the creamy appearance of your serum and bring it to someone's attention. It requires further evaluation, explanation, and management.

Lastly, I need to mention something called *lipoprotein(a)*. You guessed it—another carrier molecule. This one is a specialized form of our old friend, LDL. It's a natural occurring particle and is formed throughout the body. It's important because of the havoc it wreaks when present in elevated amounts, causing increased formation of those pesky foam cells and increasing the deposit of lipids in established atherosclerotic plaques. To top things off, it also interferes with the beneficial breaking down of clots in our blood vessels.

Some of the lipids and carriers we've been talking about are clearly associated with the development of heart disease. For example, a mountain of evidence demonstrates that elevated levels of cholesterol go hand-in-hand with the development of cardiovascular disease. While critically significant, it doesn't prove causation. There's a difference.

We are gathering consistent evidence that lipoprotein(a) *causes* heart disease. Make sure you see the difference. *Causation* is a big deal. We're going to be hearing and reading a lot more about this particle in the future—most likely the *near* future. And many leading physicians and researchers believe management of this lipoprotein holds a significant key to unlocking the best ways to detect, prevent, and treat atherosclerotic heart disease.

We'll have to wait and see, but let's hope so.

46

Give Me the Details, Doc

Biostatistics

Once again, what are we talking about here? Well, whether we realize it or not, each of us deals with some form of statistics every day. What are the chances of…? How likely is it that…? We toss a coin in the air, and what are the odds of it landing on heads or on tails? See, you know the answer to that one—50/50. But what if the question becomes, "What are the odds of getting heads six times in a row?" Now it becomes a little more difficult.

But that's nothing compared to trying to determine the chances or odds of how some treatment or medication will affect a human being or a group of human beings. Now we're talking about *bio*statistics—the application of statistics to living beings, like us.

Is this stuff important? It quickly becomes critical as we try to evaluate new medical treatments and interventions—which ones work and which ones don't. And maybe more importantly, which things actually harm us. Sounds important, but why is it so difficult?

There are several answers to this question. The first and most obvious is that we can't treat humans as we do lab mice and rats. We can't study the effects on humans *directly* as we do with these animals. We have to evaluate the effects on humans more *indirectly*, making assumptions and inferences.

For example, let's consider something called the *LD50*. This term that refers to the dose of a substance, whether a toxin or routinely used medication, at which 50 percent of people taking it would die. The 50 percent *lethal dose*. This is important when it comes to intentional and accidental overdoses, as well as the safe dose of frequently used medications. This is impossible to study in humans, given that few of us would volunteer for this kind of experiment. So we study it in lab animals and make inferences—extrapolations—and hope they are right. With that LD50 in mind, we can make human observations, not experiments, and see if we were correct in our assumptions.

But every once in a while, some terrible accident or event occurs, and we are able to study the *direct* effects of something on humans and to learn important information. The atomic bombings of Hiroshima and Nagasaki were just such terrible events. Scientists and physicians found themselves having to study the effects of sudden and massive radiation on those who survived, providing us with knowledge that we would never have been able to obtain otherwise.

What are some of the other things that make this so difficult? One important problem is something called *confounders*—literally things that perplex and bewilder. These factors confuse and distort research, making interpretation of results very difficult. Some examples of confounders are age, sex, body size, smoking habits, alcohol consumption, exercise levels, dietary habits, place of habitation, profession and educational levels, and current diseases (such as diabetes, kidney disease, heart problems, hypertension). The list goes on and on, with each of these *confounders* having a variable amount of influence on the outcome of a study.

Not so with lab mice. They can all be of the same age, all of the same sex, all given the same diet every day of their lives, most don't get past high school, and few of them smoke. Makes it a lot easier to study these critters and get useful, reproducible results. Again, not so with humans.

Here is where *biostatistics* comes into play. This field of study has given us ways to look at the outcomes of treatments and medications, adjusting for the presence of confounders and giving us useful information. It's all mathematical and headache-producing.

I discovered that the hard way. As I was pursuing a master's degree in public health at the Medical College of Wisconsin, one of the first courses I was required to pass was "Biostatistics." Looked interesting, and it started off with some basic probabilities and determinations of odds and likelihoods—useful stuff if you were going to Vegas. But the course quickly turned very difficult, requiring more study than I had imagined.

It was only after I passed the final exam that I was informed the course was considered the "rate-limiting-step" of the master's program, the threshold course that determined a student's real interest in going forward. It washed out a lot of us, and I understood why. But don't worry—we're going to talk only about broad concepts here and not multiple equations and various analyses. That's a headache now for someone else.

There are some things we need to understand. First of all, not all medical studies are created equal. Some are much better than others and give much more meaningful results. The gold standard is the "double-blinded, randomized, placebo-controlled" model. In addition to being the best, it's also the most difficult to perform. It requires that neither the study participants nor the researchers know who's in which group (the ones receiving the study medication, for example). They are all "blinded." And the participants are "randomized," meaning they are assigned to a group randomly and not chosen because of any factor such as age or sex. Lastly, the study is "placebo-controlled," meaning that the final results should be able to tell us whether a treatment or medication is better than a placebo or sugar pill. The importance of that should be obvious, but amazingly, a lot of studies don't do that. As a matter of fact, there is some guidance from the FDA that if a new drug is being studied and compared to an existing medication, it only has to be "equally effective"—not more effective, and not necessarily better than a sugar pill. Think about that for a moment.

Something else to consider about medical studies is the number of people involved. The greater the number, the more "robust" the results (a term biostatisticians like to use, meaning reliable, valid, and reproducible). There is no magical number, but you would like to have thousands of subjects in your study if you are going to draw significant conclusions.

Is all this confusing? You betcha, but it's the only way we have of studying the human response to medical interventions. And when done well, it works. But as with most things, facts can be manipulated.

More about that in the next chapter.

47

A Guide to the Latest Studies

"The latest medical studies…"

"New research has shown…"

"I just read…"

We've all heard it. Some new medical claim is made and the media floods the airwaves or Internet with the "latest and greatest" breakthrough. It quickly becomes an established fact and a talking point. Then, almost as quickly, it vaporizes, drifting off to that distant place of "What were we talking about?"

What are we to make of these life-changing discoveries? How do we deal with all the experts out there and their new research?

For the most part, take it with a grain of salt. That's an interesting idiom, and very appropriate for this issue. One theory of its origin has it that the Roman general Pompey was convinced he could become immune to being poisoned (apparently an occupational hazard at the time) by taking small amounts of various poisons along with a grain of salt. The salt apparently acted as a sort of antidote. That works here as well. Don't be "poisoned" or confused by all of the hard-to-believe claims.

You might be thinking, *But Dr. Lesslie, you've quoted some "recent research" and "medical studies" in this book. Care to explain yourself?*

That's a great question, and leads to the answer of this dilemma. I in fact *have* relied on numerous studies and research articles as background for much of this material, but I do so cautiously. There's a lot of bogus information to be found, some in places you would least expect. I think it has something to do with people wanting to be heard, to raise their hand and have someone pay attention. They just need to be sure that what they're saying or writing is substantiated by fact. That's why we spent the last two chapters looking at biostatistics and how to make some sense of the numbers thrown at us, and how to separate the wheat from the chaff.

The key here is to have confidence in your sources. As physicians, we learn where we can find reliable information, and then we have to use our experience and some measure of logic. If something is too good to be true, it probably isn't.

So what are my sources? How would I advise you to evaluate a new medical claim or look up some information for a particular illness or treatment? First of all, I'm not one to advise my patients against seeking information on the Internet. I just expect to pull up a chair and talk with my patients about the information they're finding. But blindly surfing the net will quickly lead you to some spurious info, so I *do* advise against that.

There are a few websites I can recommend with confidence. These are well-established institutions and authoritative in many areas of medical care and research. I would go here first to answer questions that may arise or to gain perspective on some medical miracle.

- www.cdc.gov—This is the CDC website, and I've referred to it on several occasions. This is no-nonsense information and there's stuff here about everything.
- www.medlineplus.gov—This is a user-friendly site with a lot of good information.
- www.mayoclinic.org—Another user-friendly site and easy to navigate.
- www.health.harvard.edu—Hey, this is Harvard. They must know what they're talking about.
- http://my.clevelandclinic.org/health/default.aspx—The Cleveland Clinic is a highly regarded institution, and I've found their website to be very useful.

These should be enough websites to help you find whatever you're looking for. Just remember when you hear some new claim or miracle breakthrough, or someone is quoting the "overwhelming evidence" of some new study, it's always wise to let the dust settle; the truth will usually find its way to the surface. (How about that for mixing metaphors.)

A grain of salt—and don't believe everything you hear. Unfortunately, Winston Churchill had it right when he said,

> "A lie gets halfway around the world
> before the truth has a chance to put its pants on."

48

When Liars Figure

Why would anyone want to manipulate the results of medical studies, something so important to each of us? The answer is simple—money. More correctly, *big* money. We're talking billions here. And if you take a prescription medication now—or might ever in the future—this affects you.

You may have heard the term "Big Pharma." This refers to the major pharmaceutical companies, of which there are many. They have a lot at stake when it comes to medical research. Their products and profitability are on the line, and if a study fails to show their medication to be of value (or worse, shows it to be potentially harmful), that flushing sound is their millions and billions going down the drain. We would like to think their main concern is to develop drugs that help alleviate some of the afflictions of the human condition—pain, suffering, disease. That may not be the case. Let me give you an example.

A category of medications—muscle relaxers—has been around for quite a while. The reality is that they probably do not in fact relax muscles but rather dull certain areas in our brain that causes the perception that something is going on. But that's not the point here. As I said, these medicines have been used for quite a while—you might have taken some yourself.

One popular medication lost its patent protection several years ago, and a couple of generics were ready to head into the market. That's generally a good thing for consumers, with generics usually costing less than the brand name. So what did the original manufacturer do? You'd think they would have made enough money with the drug while it was protected, and they'd have something new and useful in the pipeline—a different class of antibiotic or a novel treatment for one of the many diseases that still afflict us. No, they were ready with a new drug alright, but it turned out to be the old one, just at half the original dose. And the FDA gave them a whole new patent for it.

The spiel from the drug reps was that the original dose caused a lot of drowsiness, and the new reduced dose would be less sedating. It took how many years to figure that one out? And guess what? The new and improved medication costs much more than the generics and even more than the original drug.

Unfortunately, this isn't an isolated case. A waste of valuable time and opportunities, but not isolated.

Not too long ago, my medical partner found himself on a 747 bound for the West Coast. Sitting beside him was a middle-aged woman, an executive with a large pharmaceutical company. At some point she learned he was a physician, and the conversation turned to the topic of generic medications and patents. She must have assumed she had a sympathetic ear.

"Whenever we have a successful drug that is about to come off patent, we simply approach the generic manufacturers and pay them not to make our medication for a specified period of time. Our drug might be generic, but we will still be the only ones making it." (Read $$$.)

A recent exposé in the *New York Times* indicated the payment for such an agreement might be in the hundreds of millions of dollars.

It's not my intent here to bash the pharmaceutical industry—plenty of people are doing that. I believe it's important, though, to have a sense of the lay of the land. And while research is being carried out in many areas of the medical field, most of the things we hear and read about pertain to new medications. With that in mind, we need to consider the following points about that research and how it can be manipulated.

- Medical research isn't cheap, and somebody has to pay the tab. All too often, drug companies provide the needed financial support to conduct these studies, which almost always involve their own medications. This is one significant source of bias that can lead to the publishing of less than accurate results.

- The researchers who conduct these studies frequently have financial ties with these very companies. This threatens their ability to be truly objective and is a clear conflict of interest and another source of bias.

- The majority of published medical studies are positive—the drug or intervention really works, or is more effective than some other treatment, or it's even better than we thought. Negative studies—the new medicine didn't work or actually harmed those taking it—don't make it into print. Some don't even make it out of the research lab. This is really troubling and another source of bias and manipulation of the facts.

- As previously noted, results of important studies are reported in ways that are intended to be confusing—either overstating or understating the findings.

All of this makes it very difficult for those of us trying to take care of our patients. What are we to believe? Who can we rely on for objective information?

It's not all bad news here. A growing number of concerned and dedicated researchers, scientists, and physicians are turning on the lights—illuminating the dark recesses of this secretive and lucrative quagmire that has remained unchallenged for too long. The goal is for medical research to be conducted with as little bias as possible, eliminating the influence of drug companies and ensuring the utmost objectivity of the researchers. We should be able to do that.

But until that time comes, we need to remember the words of Mark Twain: "Figures can lie and liars can figure."

49

Somethin's Fishy Around Here

Fish. Now here's something we can sink our teeth into. It's not very often that we have an issue with a big upside but little if any downside. That's where we are with fish and fish-oil supplements. A couple of definitions will help, since there seems to be some confusion with the terminology.

First, we're dealing with **polyunsaturated fatty acids**—PUFAs (yes, that's actually the correct term). These are our *good* fats, essential to our health while providing substantial and multiple benefits. Then we have our omega-3 fatty acids. These are also PUFAs and are called *omega* because of the location of a certain chemical bond on their carbon chains. Sometimes this site is called the "n" location, and some researchers refer to these as n-3 PUFAs. It's all the same thing, and of these omega-3s, two are very important—EPA and DHA. You can look up their chemical names if you need to, but that's all the biochemistry for this chapter.

These fatty acids, EPA and DHA, are absorbed from our GI tract and transported to our liver. There they are bound to HDL and LDL and transported throughout our bodies, where they are incorporated into the membranes of our cells. This is where they do their beneficial work, and it can happen quickly. We are able to see changes in our cells and in our blood vessels within as little as two weeks after regularly consuming these fatty acids.

What are these benefits and how do they help us?

We know that fish oil reduces the risk of at least two fateful cardio-vascular events—death from coronary heart disease and sudden cardiac death. This reduction can occur as early as in that two-week timeframe after increasing your consumption. The mechanism apparently has to do with the PUFAs' ability to stabilize the electrical patterns in our hearts—a sudden arrhythmia is what happens with many sudden and unexpected deaths. And it doesn't take a lot of fish oil to accomplish this—less than 500 mgs a day (we'll put this into perspective a little later).

At higher levels of intake and over longer periods of time, we see an impact on several other important factors.

Blood lipid levels. Triglycerides can be lowered by as much as 25 to 30 percent. This degree of reduction requires 3 to 4 grams per day. HDL can be raised, but only a little—maybe 3 percent.

Blood pressure. Fish-oil supplementation can result in a modest lowering of both systolic and diastolic pressures. This is thought to be caused by a reduction in blood vessel stiffness.

Anti-inflammatory effects. There is some evidence that EPA and DHA both may act in this way, partly explaining their beneficial influence on arteries and existing plaque.

Heart rate. Interestingly, fish oil appears to mildly lower our resting heart rates and can stabilize "heart rate variability"—an indicator of cardiac irritability.

Heart failure. For those of us with this condition, fish oil can improve the pumping action and strength of our hearts.

Arterial wall stability. This is our *endothelium*, the inner lining of our arteries—where plaques begin and grow. Some studies have demonstrated the ability of PUFAs to improve the function of this layer and to increase the dilating capability of these vessels—an indication of blood vessel health.

Blood clotting. Higher doses of fish oil (3 to 15 grams/day) can cause unwanted bleeding. PUFAs may accomplish this through actions on our platelets, but we're not sure. Less clotting in our plaques and vessel walls is what we want, and fish oil seems to help with this without causing any significant bleeding elsewhere, even with those taking Coumadin or other blood thinners.

Atherosclerosis. Several studies of the effects of PUFAs have demonstrated a reduction in the formation of new plaques and a slowing of the growth of existing ones.

Sudden cardiac death and death due to coronary heart disease. We mentioned this before, but this is the important stuff and warrants being repeated. With only minimally increased amounts of daily fish oil (estimated to be 250 to 500 mgs of DHA and EPA), we see a reduction in these deaths by as much as 36 percent. That's a lot, and reason enough to pay attention to our intake of fish and fish oil.

That's a lot of upside. Now, about the downside.

Hmm...not much here. The most common problems are GI complaints, usually nausea, and only in a small percentage of patients. Other than this occasional stomach upset, the most common complaint we hear with supplements is that they create a fishy taste, especially after a person belches. This can be helped by freezing the capsule, taking it with a meal, or both. And regarding the potential for bleeding, this side effect has seldom been demonstrated with doses up to 4 grams/day—more than enough fish oil to accomplish all the above actions. So, PUFAs are safe.

If you're convinced, as I am, that PUFAs—especially from fish oil— are something we need to increase in our diets, how do we go about doing that?

The first and maybe the best opportunity is to increase our intake of fish. But not just *any* fish. All of the studies refer to the "oily" varieties, those that provide high levels of omega-3 fatty acids. For comparative reasons, I've listed various types of fish with the number of three-and-a-half-ounce servings required to achieve a daily intake of 250 mg of DHA and EPA—the threshold amount needed to prevent sudden cardiac deaths.

- Atlantic salmon—one serving
- canned anchovies—one
- Atlantic herring—one
- Atlantic mackerel—two
- bluefin tuna—two
- rainbow trout—two
- striped bass—two (this surprised me)
- canned sardines—two

White or nonoily fish includes the following:

- sea bass—three

- snapper—six
- flounder and sole—six
- light canned tuna—seven
- grouper—eight
- catfish—eight
- Atlantic cod—twelve

That's a wide range and a lot of canned tuna to eat in order to meet the daily goal of 250 mgs. Fortunately, there are many over-the-counter fish oil preparations and a few prescription formulations. That makes it easier, but we still have to pay attention and make sure we read those labels. The amounts of EPA and DHA can vary significantly among preparations, so check this out before buying. If the goal is to reduce your chances of sudden death, 1 gram (1,000 mgs) a day is all you'll need—actually more than enough. If you're trying to reduce an elevated triglyceride level, we're looking at 3 to 4 grams a day. Still safe, but you don't want to go any higher without talking with your physician.

So there you are. Unless there's a medical reason not to do so, all of us need to add fish oil to our daily diets.

50

Don't Be Mislabeled: Making Sense of Those Nutritional Numbers

Reading nutritional food labels may not be as enjoyable as reading a *New York Times* bestseller, but you just might learn some interesting things, improve your and your family's health, and if done correctly, *not* tick off the store manager.

That's right—there's an acceptable way to do this and a way... Well, I'll just give you some advice. My wife suggested I use my smartphone to gather information for this chapter. Simply take some pictures of labels and study them at home at my leisure. Not going to happen. It seems most if not all grocery stores frown upon shoppers taking pictures. Take my word for this and don't try it. I was glad I had a clipboard with pre-printed info sheets and could study boxes and cans and make notes of all the numbers. It was a little cumbersome, and I still had some 'splainin' to do to the store manager. But it worked.

Before I share some of the things I learned, let's take a look at a "nutritional food label" and try to understand what information it contains. The Food and Drug Administration has a great website for this at www.fda.gov/Food/IngredientsPackagingLabeling/LabelingNutrition/ucm274593.htm. Below is one of their examples and a good place to begin.

Nutrition Facts

Serving Size 2/3 cup (55g)
Servings Per Container About 8

Amount Per Serving

Calories 230   Calories from Fat 72

	% Daily Value*
Total Fat 8g	**12%**
Saturated Fat 1g	**5%**
Trans Fat 0g	
Cholesterol 0mg	**0%**
Sodium 160mg	**7%**
Total Carbohydrate 37g	**12%**
Dietary Fiber 4g	**16%**
Sugars 1g	
Protein 3g	

Vitamin A	10%
Vitamin C	8%
Calcium	20%
Iron	45%

* Percent Daily Values are based on a 2,000 calorie diet.
Your daily value may be higher or lower depending on
your calorie needs.

	Calories:	2,000	2,500
Total Fat	Less than	65g	80g
Sat Fat	Less than	20g	25g
Cholesterol	Less than	300mg	300mg
Sodium	Less than	2,400mg	2,400mg
Total Carbohydrate		300g	375g
Dietary Fiber		25g	30g

Let's start with "Serving Size." This is really important and frequently overlooked. It can be tricky, and I've misread this myself, on more than one occasion. In this example, the serving size is 2/3 of a cup. It's worth the time to take out a measuring cup and see how much we're talking about. If it's breakfast cereal, I bet you're eating a lot more than 2/3 of a cup. The tricky part for me is when the serving size is given in ounces or teaspoons or tablespoons. You have to pay attention. These sizes make a big difference in calorie counts, fat grams, and carbs.

Let's go to "Calories." This is straightforward, but you have to remember the serving size. If this example is for a breakfast cereal and you're eating two cups of it, that's more than twice the amount of calories listed.

Simple math, but you have to pay attention. As for the "Calories from Fat," you don't have to pay much attention to this if you're on a low-carb diet.

While we're talking about calories, here's a sobering thought. It's generally accepted that if you take in 3,000 more calories than you burn, you will gain one pound. In other words, you have to burn 3,000 calories to lose one pound. Twenty minutes on a treadmill at 3.7 mph at an incline of 5 degrees burns about 150 calories. One 12-ounce can of regular soda contains 140 calories. Go figure.

Now we move on to "Total Fat." This area of the label breaks down the fat content of a product. This particular label lists only saturated fat and trans fat, while others will break it down further to tell us how much of the total fat is mono or polyunsaturated. The trans-fat number here is 0 grams, which is good. This type of fat should be disappearing from the US marketplace. Bear in mind that the FDA does not require listing an amount if the trans-fat content is less than 0.5 grams in a serving, so this unnatural and deadly grease can still be present and add up. For the most part, take the "Total Fat" and subtract the "Saturated" variety. That leaves us with the unsaturated and healthier kinds. Remember, we need to work on reducing the saturated fat in our diets.

Next we see the "Cholesterol" content of this food. We should limit this in our diets, but keep in mind it's not so much the cholesterol we take in that drives up the level in our body. It's several factors, including our individual genetic makeup, the amount of carbs we eat, and the amount of exercise we get.

The "Sodium" (salt) content is important for all of us, especially if our blood pressure is high or even borderline. Actually, *all* of us need to limit this mineral because of its harmful effects. That's difficult, because it finds its way into many of our processed foods. The American Heart Association currently recommends an intake of less than 1500 mgs/day. With our example, you can see how this adds up.

Now the "Total Carbohydrate" numbers. This is where we really need to pay attention. The low-carb approach targets 60 grams as a limit. I think this number can be bumped to 100, but as you can see, this example shows 37 grams. That's typical for a lot of cereals, breads, and other processed grains. And with only one serving, you're well on your way to the daily max.

"Dietary Fiber" is important, and remember the recommended daily amount of 25 grams for women and 38 for men. Most nutrition experts refer to "net carbs." This is calculated by subtracting the fiber amount from the total carbohydrates. (Some recommend subtracting half of the fiber.) The more fiber in a food, the lower its glycemic index and the less impact it will have on your blood sugar.

Next we see "Sugars." This is the total amount of natural sugars (as found in fruit and milk, for example) along with any added sugars. It's the added ones you need to pay attention to, and these can be found in the "Ingredients" section, which usually appears on product packaging somewhere near the "Nutrition Facts." Added sugars can include corn syrup, high-fructose corn syrup, fruit juice concentrate, maltose, dextrose, sucrose, and even honey and maple syrup. All of these add carbs to our diet and are largely unneeded.

A couple of points: When we study these food labels, we're probably holding in our hands something processed—something we need to eliminate as much as possible from our diets. And the ingredients list on a food label works just like the ingredients list on a pet food label—contents are listed in descending order by weight. Something to keep in mind for you and your pet.

The amount of "Protein" listed is just that and is of concern if you have to limit your intake, usually because of significant kidney problems. It's also of interest because of the places you find—or don't find—this essential building block.

That leaves us with the percentage of recommended daily allowances for various vitamins and minerals. I don't pay much attention to this since it really doesn't enter into my equation for determining the healthiness of a particular food. For instance, in our example, you would have to eat almost 7 cups of this stuff to achieve 100 percent of your daily vitamin A needs. Yet, you may find this information interesting.

Now that we have a handle on reading a nutritional label, brace yourselves—the FDA is proposing to revise it. You can find an example on the FDA website listed earlier in this chapter, and it actually makes a lot of sense. The important things are emphasized and the not-so-important are minimized.

I mentioned my fact-finding trip to the grocery store. In addition to learning that cameras aren't allowed, I found the following to be of interest:

- A lot of us eat salads and salad dressings. All of these dressings contain fats, but mostly of the healthy kind. You have to watch the amounts (most list 2 tablespoons as one serving) so the calories can quickly add up. The lowest in carb content are blue cheese (1 gram per serving) followed by ranch (1 to 2 grams).

- You have to pay attention to the "lite" dressings. Sounds healthy, but they take out some of the fat and add a lot of sugar. Some of these have 16 to 18 grams/serving.

- All of our breakfast cereals are loaded with carbs, and many have added sugars—especially those we feed to our children.

- Check the sugar contents of "healthy" and "all-natural" fruit drinks. And bring your insulin.

- As a general rule, anything labeled "all-natural" should be carefully scrutinized.

Make it a habit to read those labels. And remember, "If it comes in a can, box, wrapper, or through a fast-food window, it's probably going to eventually kill you."

51

Vitamin D and Your Heart

It seems our old friend vitamin D has become somewhat of a superstar. The past few years have seen an expanding array of healthcare claims for this essential nutrient, and the list continues to grow.

In addition to its well-established role in bone and muscle health, some of those claims include a reduction in the risk of developing certain cancers (colon, breast, prostate, esophageal, and ovarian) as well as diabetes. Other assertions are that it can help lower blood pressure, reduce the incidence of colon polyps, reduce the risk of falling, slow or maybe prevent the onset of dementia, and possibly reduce the incidence of multiple sclerosis. Most recently we have read of its positive impact on our hearts. If all or most of these are valid, vitamin D truly is a superstar.

But what do we really know? Not as much as we think or hope. We probably know more about what a *deficiency* of this vitamin looks like. Rickets is one of those problems, and it causes slowed growth and deformities of our long bones (arms and legs). This is another of the diseases we study about but don't see in this country. Other boney problems include osteomalacia (a thinning of the bones with associated fractures and muscle weakness) and osteoporosis (reduced bone mineral density, also associated with bone weakness and fractures). Muscle twitching and weakness, as well as lightheadedness have been well-described. These conditions respond to the correction of low vitamin D levels, thus supporting the principle of cause and effect.

We're comfortable with our understanding of the importance of this nutrient for our bone and muscle health. What about these other health claims?

That's where things become a little less solid. Many of these theories are based on *observational studies,* which we've discussed earlier. Interesting, but lacking in rigorous, thorough research. The best evidence seems to support the benefits of vitamin D for slowing the development and worsening of dementia, including Alzheimer's disease. If this bears fruit, that would be cause for great rejoicing. And since these are such profound and life-altering diseases, *any* beneficial effect, no matter how small, would be welcomed. That's true for a lot of the problems we face today—any help, any small step forward will be happily embraced.

What about the connection between this vitamin and our hearts? Or with our lipid levels? Here's what we know.

People with high blood pressure, heart failure, and other cardiovascular diseases (strokes, heart attacks) *tend* to have lower vitamin D levels than those who don't have these problems. Additionally, as levels of vitamin D go down, we see more hypertension and more obesity (especially the central variety, with the disproportionately large waistline we've previously discussed).

All of these problems tend to improve as our vitamin D levels go up. The operative word here is *tend,* meaning current evidence points in that direction, but we await large and ongoing clinical trials to really know for sure.

Regarding our lipid levels, a large randomized study (remember, this is much better than the observational type) demonstrated that in a group of women who received vitamin D supplementation, an increase in their vitamin D levels was associated with a small but important reduction in their LDL. This is significant and may help to explain the benefits of this nutrient for our hearts and vascular systems.

Who's at risk of being vitamin D deficient? And what do we do about it?

The first step is to have your blood tested and determine your level. In our clinic, we see people of all ages, colors, and sizes, and we check a lot of vitamin D levels. Of all those we test, 60 to 70 percent are vitamin D deficient.

It has long been held that since most of our active vitamin D (D_3) is formed in our skin, those of us receiving plenty of sunshine (below a latitude of 40° N) shouldn't have anything to worry about. We live near Charlotte and get a lot of sunshine (a latitude of 35°13'3" N for those who are counting), so something else is going on here.

The reality is that the amount of sunshine we get must not be the key factor. We see farmers with leathered, sun-damaged skin whose levels are low, and pale office workers whose levels are well within the normal range. Yet we know that complications of many cardiovascular diseases occur more frequently during the winter months, when there is less sunshine and vitamin D levels are the lowest. And mounting evidence suggests the onset of type 2 diabetes is more common among those of us with low levels and less sun exposure.

It's a conundrum, wrapped in a mystery, inside an enigma. But it seems clear that our individual amount of daily sunshine is not the complete answer. Dietary intake is going to be just as important if not more so.

So with these points in mind, we have our level tested and it's low. How did that happen?

There are many risk factors for having a low level. If it's because of a decreased production in the skin due to inadequate sun exposure (not enough UV radiation), this can be due to being older, having covered or colored skin, living in an area where there is limited and less-direct sunshine, being obese, or just choosing to avoid the sun altogether. If low vitamin D level is caused by a lack of dietary vitamin D, this is more often found with vegetarians, vegans, women, those who have had various stomach surgeries, and those suffering with various food allergies.

That's a long list, and may help to explain why so many of our patients are deficient. The good news is that this can easily be corrected. While paying attention to what we eat and trying to increase the amounts of vitamin D in our diets, keep in mind vegetables and fruits contain little of this nutrient. The best sources are cod liver oil, bacon, salmon, oysters, sardines, and egg yolks. Not much to choose from if you're a vegetarian—maybe not much to choose from for the rest of us. Most will need to find another source. Fortunately, many OTC supplements are available, and most are inexpensive. A good starting point is to add 1,000 to 2,000 units of D_3 to your diet. The D_3 designation is critical, since this is the active form of vitamin D.

"But Doc, I take a multivitamin with D in it. Shouldn't that be enough?"

Check the label. The answer is no. The amounts are usually in the low to mid hundreds, and we need more than that. It's difficult to overdose on this vitamin, and 2,000 units should be safe for most. Talk to your physician before taking more.

We're going to learn more in the coming years about this important vitamin, and our approach to dealing with it may change. While vitamin D won't cure baldness, improve your love life, or give you sudden and magical insight into dealing with your teenage children, it *will* help your bones and muscles.

And there's a very good chance it will also help with your lipid levels and the health of your heart.

52

You Gotta Know Your Numbers

Too Soon

Paige Carson rubbed her stomach and continued staring at the computer screen. She was reading about gallbladder disease and decided her symptoms fit the description presented on a popular healthcare website.

I've got to get this checked out. Maybe tomorrow.

The pain had been getting worse and more frequent. But what bothered her was the left arm pain. That was new.

The twenty-seven-year-old closed her laptop, double-laced her running shoes, and headed out into the cool of the early morning and her daily five-mile run.

"Let's see, Miss Carson." Bruce Evans, the newest physician in one of the largest family-practice groups in town, was studying Paige's chart. "I see that you've been having some epigastric pain—upper abdominal, I believe you note. And you're concerned about possible gallbladder problems."

He moved to the chair beside her exam table and sat down. Evans was young, only four or five years older than Paige. This was the first time they had seen each other, and he was rapidly thumbing through her slender medical file. She didn't get sick very often.

"That's right, Doctor. I'm wondering if this pain has something to do with my gallbladder, but mainly I just want to know what it is and what I need to do to make it go away."

"I'm sure you do. That's my job—to find an answer and try to fix it."

She caught herself glancing at the door and wondering where Dr. Winters might be. The older family physician had always taken care of her and knew the family history.

"Everything here looks fine," Evans said, turning a few more pages in her file. "No recent lab work, though. Looks like it's been two, maybe three years since we checked things." He paused and leaned closer to the chart. "Hmm. Your cholesterol…It was a little high back then. Almost 250. And your HDL—your good cholesterol—was very low. Have the doctors here had you on any medicine for that?"

Paige shook her head. "No, I've never been on any medication, except for birth-control pills. But our family has—"

Bruce Evans closed the chart and tossed it onto the nearby countertop. "We can address that at some point in the future—repeat your labs and all. But I don't think that cholesterol has any bearing on the discomfort you've been experiencing. It's a risk factor for cardiac disease, as you know, but if you're concerned about your heart, don't be. You're young, slender, active, and a female. All of that is working in your favor. Now tell me some more about this pain you've been having."

Paige absently rubbed her left arm and glanced at her medical record. *Did he even look at the family history part? Did he notice that my dad died at the age of thirty-nine and my thirty-two-year-old brother already has three stents in his coronary arteries?*

"Miss Carson?"

She looked up at Bruce Evans. He was tapping the end of his pen on the countertop.

"Yes, I'm sorry. What was the question?"

"I was asking about your abdominal pain. Are there things that make it worse? Different kinds of food or drinking alcohol? Or anything that seems to relieve it?"

"No, I've read about that, and I've paid close attention to what I eat. Nothing special seems to bring it on—no greasy foods or things like that. And I don't drink."

He made some notes on the chart.

"I see. And what makes it better? Do you take anything for it, such as antacids or something like that?"

"I've tried several over-the-counter stomach medicines, but it usually just goes away when I sit down and try to relax."

"Hmm." Evans made more notes and nodded his head.

There were more questions, followed by a brief physical exam.

"Not typical for gallbladder disease," he said. "But I think it needs to be ruled out. We'll get you scheduled for an ultrasound later on this week and see what that shows. In the meantime, I want you to pay close attention to when this pain occurs, what you're doing when it starts, and try to remember what you've eaten before it happens. That would all be very helpful."

Evans stood up and stepped to the door. "Any questions at this point?"

Paige sighed and shook her head. "Let's just hope the ultrasound gives us the answer. I'm just ready for this to go away."

He smiled and tucked his pen into his coat pocket. "I'm sure you are, Miss Carson. We'll find the answer. And don't worry, we'll take care of whatever it is."

The door closed behind him, and Paige was alone, blankly staring at the tiled floor.

"Well, it doesn't seem to be your gallbladder." Bruce Evans had called Paige at home, giving her the negative results of her ultrasound. "Completely normal. No stones or thickening of the wall. It's all clear."

There was silence as Paige considered this information. She hadn't wanted surgery, but she desperately wanted an answer. The pain seemed to be getting worse and more frequent. It had awakened her early this morning—about 3:00 a.m.—and she hadn't been able to get back to sleep.

"I think what we'll need to do, Miss Carson, is bring you in for some lab work. We'll start from scratch and see what we can find. I've talked with Dr. Winters about your case, and he informed me about your family history, from a cardiac standpoint. Early heart disease, I believe. But again, you're a young, healthy woman, and I don't believe that's what we're dealing with. Just to be safe, though, we'll check things out, starting with those labs."

"Okay, Dr. Evans. I think I can come by in the morning, if that works."

"That will be fine. I'll make sure my nurse knows you're coming, and what studies she needs to draw. We'll see you then."

Paige Carson never had her blood drawn, and she never made it to Dr. Evans's office. She died on a deserted sidewalk while jogging—her heart quivering helplessly, its blood supply suddenly cut off by coronary arteries filled with cholesterol plaques.

"If you're concerned about your heart, don't be."

53

Your Momma Was Right:
Eat Your Fruits and Vegetables

Most of us probably don't have to be convinced that fruits and vegetables are good for us. That's overwhelmingly true, but there can be a few pitfalls.

Let's start with how much of these we should be eating each day. The Centers for Disease Control (CDC) has a great website for this, as well as other areas of nutritional interest. You can check it out at www.cdc.gov/nutrition/everyone/fruitsvegetables.

Most nutritionists now agree that five seems to be the magic number. We need five servings of fruits and vegetables each day, with some from each group. Any combination is fine, and the more the merrier. A serving can be a little tricky (the CDC site will help with this), but generally one cup equals one serving. With fruit, for instance, one serving would be one cup of 100 percent fruit juice, one cup of sliced or chopped fruit, one small apple or banana or orange or peach. That doesn't seem like a lot, but we have to plan a little and make sure we're getting enough.

When it comes to these foods, they're not all created equal. Some are much better for us than others, and some should generally be avoided. Don't throw any rotten tomatoes at me, but we should be eating little if any pineapple (way too much sugar) and bananas (also way too much sugar). Check out the carb counts if you don't believe me, keeping in mind that a low-carb diet targets 60 grams of carbs a day as the threshold. (I'll go ahead and tell you—27 grams in a banana and 22 in one cup of pineapple.)

And speaking of tomatoes, it doesn't matter how you pronounce it—*a rose by any other name*—it's technically a fruit and a nutritional powerhouse. We'll talk more about that in a moment. Right now, let's consider the health benefits of fruits and vegetables.

Several large studies have demonstrated lower blood pressures in individuals consuming 5-plus servings/day when compared with those who eat less. There is also evidence that LDL is reduced in this same group, though this effect is not large. Yet we see less cardiovascular disease in these people, though it may be due to several factors. For instance, we know that fruits and vegetables:

- contain a variety of potent antioxidants
- are our main source of fiber, with its associated benefits
- provide a wide array of vitamins and minerals
- add color to our meals (that's actually important and we'll see why)

I mentioned a few pitfalls, and we've looked at bananas and pineapples—a couple of our high-sugar friends. We also need to pay attention to the amount of legumes on our plates. These would be our beans, peas, and even peanuts. If it's starchy, it probably contains a lot of carbs. Navy beans, pintos, peas, black beans—these are the starchy varieties. They contain a lot of good things, such as fiber, vitamins, and proteins. But though their carbs are slowly digested, they still considerably add to our carb load. This is important to each of us, especially those with diabetes or a predisposition to developing it.

Green beans contain fewer carbohydrates, as do green leafy vegetables, broccoli, asparagus, cauliflower, and many others. This is important to know, and easy-to-use information tables are readily accessible on the Internet. (The CDC site is also a great source for this.) For a little perspective, here's some comparisons. We'll include a few of our starchy vegetables and really sweet fruits:

Carbohydrates (in grams) found in one serving:

- baked potato—60
- sweet potato—60

- corn on the cob—30-45
- legumes/lentils—15
- apple—15
- dried prunes—15
- dates—15
- strawberries—12
- carrots—5
- raw leafy vegetables—3
- broccoli—3
- cauliflower—3
- asparagus—2
- mushrooms—1/2 (You're right—this is not a fruit or a vegetable.)

This gives us an idea of the carb counts of some commonly encountered fruits and vegetables. I'm not advising that we preoccupy ourselves with this—just be aware of it, especially if you decide to lower your overall carb intake.

Now for some fun. Let's take a look at a few of our interesting foods and what they can do for us.

Broccoli. Well, it might not be *that* interesting, but broccoli does a lot of good things for us. It's a great source of vitamin C and folic acid as well as several important antioxidants. And it's a good source of fiber. The key is to not overcook it; eating it raw or steamed is best.

Avocado. This is one of our few fatty fruits, and it contains a lot of calories (330) and fat (30 grams). But it's the good kind of fat and can actually reduce our cholesterol level. This is an important component of the South Beach and Mediterranean diets, so something good must be going on here. We know it's an important source of vitamins C and E, and glutathione—one of our body's most important antioxidants and detoxifiers. Just be careful of the calories.

Grapes. We've incorporated grapes into our diets for thousands of years. They're a good source of vitamins A, C, B_6, and folate, as well as the minerals magnesium, selenium, and potassium. Now it seems we're mainly interested in the antioxidants we find in this fruit. These include the phenolic acids, flavonoids, and resveratrol—all of which are found mainly in the skins.

Strawberries. These berries, along with blueberries and blackberries, are a great source of several vitamins as well as potent antioxidants. In addition, they are low in calories and high in fiber, making them an important addition to any diet.

Tomatoes. Earlier I referred to this fruit as a nutritional powerhouse and it is. It's one of our best sources of lycopene, another of our antioxidants with the purported ability to protect against certain types of cancer. Tomatoes contain several important vitamins as well and are an important part of the Mediterranean Diet. One easy way to incorporate these into your daily routine is the use of tomato juice or V8 (the low-salt variety). V8 has the added benefit of providing two servings of fruit and vegetables to your diet, with very few calories.

Goji berries. I need some help here. Goji berries are now the rage, with claims that they are loaded with antioxidants, few calories, and a lot of fiber. The Chinese have been eating these for more than six thousand years, and they claim they can help your liver, kidneys, vision, and circulation. The Chinese have been around for a long time, so they must know what they're talking about. In fact, several studies support many of these claims.

My problem: I'm able to grow goji berries here in South Carolina, but I have no idea what to do with them when they're ripe. I've tried eating them off the bush, but that doesn't work. They taste terrible. My plants are thriving, so I'm going to have a lot of these elongated red berries next summer. If you've got any ideas, please contact me through my blog (http://robertlesslie.com/blog).

Once more, your momma was right. Vegetables and fruits are good for us, and we should be getting at least five servings a day. This is one of those infrequent instances where more is actually good for you.

Oh, I almost forgot. I mentioned the issue of color with these foods. In addition to providing interest to our dinner plates, the many colors of our fruits and vegetables are associated with specific nutrients.

- *Red*—lycopene and other antioxidants (beets, cherries, tomatoes, pomegranates, strawberries)

- *Purple and blue*—lutein, resveratrol, vitamin C, flavonoids (blackberries, blueberries, grapes, purple cabbage, plums)
- *Orange and yellow*—beta-carotene, lycopene, flavonoids, vitamin C (carrots, oranges, peaches, grapefruit, cantaloupe, butternut squash)
- *Green*—fiber, folate, calcium, vitamin C (broccoli, spinach, peas, cabbage, lettuce, everything my grandchildren don't like)

So the color of food is important and can be fun.

By now you should be hungry. Just remember what your momma said.

54

Are You Taking Your Medicine?

I always become a little troubled when I read a report about how many prescriptions go unfilled. It doesn't make much sense, does it? Someone takes the time to seek the advice of their physician, and then they don't follow through and do their part. I understand that we all forget to take our medicine from time to time, but to never fill it in the first place? Beats me.

How often do you think this happens? We have some good information here, so take a guess. One in a hundred? One in fifty? How about one out of every three. That's right—one third of all prescriptions go unfilled. That's an amazing number. Why does it happen? And is it even important?

Let's deal with the important part first. Of course, medication can't help us if it's still in the bottle, or worse yet, still in the pharmacy. And depending on the condition, failure to receive the proper medicine can have disastrous effects—infections such as pneumonia are a glaring example. Lack of treatment for multiple and chronic diseases can lead to an increase in ER visits, more frequent hospitalizations, and even death.

Another increasingly important factor is our aging population. More of us are becoming elderly and we're living longer. Here's some unsettling information: the average Medicare patient with *one* chronic disease (such as diabetes, heart disease, kidney failure, emphysema) sees four different physicians each year. For those with five or more of these conditions, that number rises to fourteen. Fourteen different physicians each year! That raises the potential for a lot of prescriptions, and that requires a lot of coordination and communication. No wonder so many prescriptions go unfilled, even though they may be much needed.

Remember, that number is one in three. It's technically called *nonadherence* and indicates a failure to fill a prescription within nine months. That's plenty of time to get down to the corner drugstore. But all prescriptions are not created equal. Some fall into the nonadherence column more than others.

Which class of medications do you think are most often *filled*? If you answered pain medicine, you'd be right. But you might be surprised at where some of our other pharmaceutical treatments fall. For instance, the most frequently *unfilled* medications are those prescribed for ischemic heart disease (angina)—a startling one in two never make it to the pharmacy. How about thyroid replacement meds? That's also about one in two. And cardiovascular drugs? These would be blood-pressure medicines, statins, and anticoagulants, among others. One in three—our overall average.

Again, pain medicines are the most frequently filled, but after that are the antibiotics. This is especially true for those medications used to treat urinary tract infections (UTI); only one in five go unfilled. I've treated a lot of women in the ER at two in the morning with UTI symptoms, and I understand their desire for rapid and effective relief.

These are our unfilled prescription numbers, but why does it happen? As with most healthcare problems, the answer is complex and multifactored.

The high cost of many medicines stands out as the most frequent barrier to filling a prescription. The higher the cost, the more the nonadherence. But that's not the only reason. This is where things become a little confusing. If a person has recently been in the hospital, they are less likely to have a prescription filled. And the more serious their condition—unstable heart disease, difficult-to-control diabetes—the less likely also. It doesn't make much sense, but that's what the research tells us. Those are problems, but also opportunities.

If, for whatever reason, you find yourself reluctant to fill a prescription, talk with your physician. If it's a financial concern, let them know. There may be less expensive medications out there that are able to get the job done. The statins are a great example. And several programs are available for financial assistance with your pharmacy needs. Talk with your physician, or better yet his nurse, about this. Discount coupons are available, and several drug companies have cost-assistance programs.

If it's an issue of confusion about your prescription ("Do I really need to take this?"), ask for an explanation, and keep asking until you're satisfied with the answer.

Most physicians give a lot of thought before writing a prescription. What's the best medicine for my patient? What's the outcome we're trying to achieve? Will it cause more harm than good? Will she be able to afford it?

Some of these questions can be difficult to answer. But one thing's for certain—your medication won't do either of us any good if it stays in the bottle.

55

This Plaque Business: Can It Be Reversed?

This is an important question, and we would all like the answer to be a resounding yes! Unfortunately, we're not there yet, but we're on the way. Developing evidence suggests that some of this disease process can, in fact, be reversed, but it takes effort. To understand why this is so difficult to accomplish, we need to quickly review how plaques form.

We are born with pristine, clean-as-a-whistle arteries. The innermost lining—the endothelium—is smooth, healthy, and elastic. We go downhill from there.

At an early age (frequently in our teens) we begin to form atheromatous plaques—hardening of our arteries. This starts when the endothelium is damaged in some way. Current theories hold that this is most often due to high blood pressure, elevated levels of cholesterol—including LDL and triglycerides—and cigarette smoking.

(I must digress for a moment here and state that throughout my decades in the ER and in our clinic, I have too often witnessed the ravages of this senseless, killing, smoking habit. Had Dante known of the Tobacco Institute, there would have been ten circles in his *Inferno*.)

Back to our endothelium. Once damaged, several things start to happen. This can occur quickly, but it usually takes a few decades to fully develop. In an effort to heal the wound, specific cell types migrate to the vessel wall. These are platelets and macrophages, among others, and they serve a purpose. But then cholesterol and LDL become deposited, as well as other cellular debris and crystals of calcium. The plaque grows in size, with more cells and more cholesterol. As the process matures, connective tissue can work its way into this mess, acting to stabilize it, while at the same time making it very difficult for the plaque to shrink or disappear.

At this point, two things can happen—both of them bad. A piece of this plaque can break off, carried by our bloodstream to some smaller vessel where it becomes lodged, blocking the flow of blood beyond it. And you have your stroke or heart attack. This is why we want our plaques to be stable, not angry and prone to breaking apart. Our antioxidants help with this, and those free radicals we discussed earlier aggravate things.

The other potential bad thing is that something triggers the formation of a clot on the surface of the plaque, and this grows until it obstructs the entire vessel. Again, you have your stroke or heart attack. This is where blood-thinners come into play, even our lowly baby aspirin. We don't want this clot to form or grow.

So there's our plaque, and in order for this process to be reversed and for these lesions to go away, several things need to happen.

We need to see plaque stabilization but without too much of the connective tissue component. We need to reverse whatever has caused the endothelial damage and dysfunction. And we need to decrease the tendency for clot formation. These factors will allow for the removal of cholesterol, LDL, and other fats from the plaque, as well as that cellular debris and calcium. This would potentially cause it to shrink.

That's a tall order, but would have far-reaching benefits for many of us—or most of us as we grow older.

That's why I found the results of the SATURN study to be fascinating. This large, randomized study, completed only a few years ago, compared two of our statins—atorvastatin (Lipitor) and rosuvastatin (Crestor)—to determine if plaque progression could be slowed. They used the maximum doses possible, something that most physicians don't often do, and studied the coronary vessels of the study participants. This was done with an initial heart catheterization and follow-up intravascular ultrasounds. The study lasted for two years, during which time LDL levels markedly dropped—many to below 70 mg/dl—and HDL levels rose to around 50.

The researchers were able to demonstrate that these drugs at these doses slowed the progression of plaques, and in almost two thirds of the study patients were able to *reverse* the atherosclerosis. That's right—reverse it.

This is big news, but we have to temper our enthusiasm. Not everyone in the study was able to achieve these impressive reductions in their LDL, and not everyone demonstrated this reversal on their ultrasounds. Yet, the overall results are very encouraging. This study altered my practice in that I try to get my patients' LDL levels as low as possible—targeting that 70 threshold as it seems that's where good things start to happen. It takes higher doses of these statins, and we have to expect more side effects. But if we can reverse this process, we need to do whatever it takes—safely.

So the answer to this question is yes, we are learning how to improve the health of our blood vessels and reverse the damage that's been done. We're making progress.

But until we have a gently acting Drano for our blood vessels, the emphasis needs to remain on prevention. We need to make aggressive lifestyle changes, including weight loss, dietary changes, exercise, and smoking cessation. And we need to aggressively lower our lipid levels, remembering that "no LDL level is too low."

If you know you have heart disease, talk with your doctor and put it in reverse.

It's All About Balance

The sweet spot. We're all searching for it—some without realizing.

If you play golf, you know it instantly. You make contact with the ball and it's…perfect. All you've ever tried to do with a golf club has come together in this one moment, this one swing. You don't need to look up—you know where that round white object is headed.

The same is true for a tennis player. Racket meets ball and you just know. All of your power and accuracy come together in that one rare instant. Perfect.

And there's the four-part a cappella singing group. The musical piece flows to a critical moment and there it is—a chord whose harmony stirs your very soul, resonates within your entire being, transports you out of this everyday world. It doesn't matter whether you're one of the singers or someone in the audience. It's perfect.

And then reality. We stand over that golf ball, swing as hard as we can, and watch a duck hook fly out of bounds. We swing our tennis racket too early and at the wrong angle, and that fuzzy ball sails over the fence. And the baritone, approaching that climactic harmony, is suddenly moved to pursue his own unwritten musical line, and our teeth are instantly set on edge.

The sweet spot. Forever sought after. Forever elusive.

We seek that same elusive sweet spot in our lives as well. We live in an age of distraction, constantly bombarded by an ever-expanding array of diversions. Those distractions make it very difficult if not impossible for us to focus on the things and people and moments that are important. It's an internal struggle as well. Our attention is fractured by ever-shifting hopes and dreams, plans and schemes, inward hurts and wild imaginings.

We're a jumbled mess, aren't we?

Should we ever find this *balance*, what would it look like? As are many of us, I'm a visual learner—you know, "one picture is worth a thousand words." I've attached some diagrams in an attempt to convey how this might appear in our lives. It's never this simple, but we need to start somewhere.

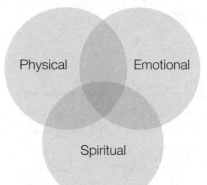

You'll note the three areas here. Let's talk about these.

The *physical* part of our lives is just that. This is largely what we deal with in our medical clinic every day—injuries, illnesses, or the desire for better health and disease prevention. We focus on what we can see and feel, and that's not a bad thing. We *need* to stay as healthy as we can for as long as we can, and to heal as quickly as possible when injured or sick. And we need to pay attention to things that can adversely affect our health, such as elevated lipid levels.

All of this is important and it's okay. It's when this area of our lives becomes unbalanced that things go wrong. We focus too much on our bodies or on how we look, or we become preoccupied with some vague symptoms that must be the first signs of a terminal illness. That circle grows larger and overwhelms the other two. In the following illustration, you can see how we can easily become detached from our spiritual being, completely obsessed with our bodies and health.

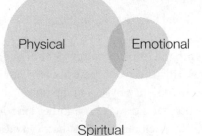

This brings us to our *emotional* part. We are certainly passionate and sensitive creatures. I've lived with two teenage daughters, and the emotional roller coaster was like Disney's Space Mountain but at twice the speed—up, down, sideways, and most of it in the dark. Anyway, some experts liken this to a colorful, interconnected cluster of feelings: love, pity, outrage, affection, happiness, suffering, self-confidence, shyness, anger, guilt, depression, pride, despair, regret, surprise, wonder, and many more. No wonder we're all over the place. It's easy to imagine how our emotional lives can quickly become distorted and out of balance.

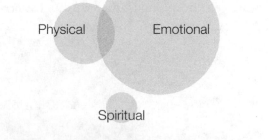

We are all too easily overwhelmed by grief and anger, blinded by love, or diminished by shyness and disappointment. We know our emotional life impacts our physical being—weight gain or loss, lack of energy, obsession with real and imagined diseases. And we know the effects too much stress can have on our health. It's a very real contributor to heart attacks and strokes, in addition to being the cause of inexplicable aches, pains, and multiple complaints. We've even seen how this chronic stress can raise our lipid levels and promote the formation of dangerous plaques in our arteries.

When our emotional lives are not in balance, bad things happen. We see it every day.

That leaves us with the *spiritual* component of our lives. What are we talking about here? This is that deepest place in our innermost beings, separate yet connected to our physical and emotional selves. It's not just a feel-good spot—that would make it another emotion. It's something altogether different. It's been described as that void created within us that longs to be filled by our Creator. Most of us would call this our *soul*. C.S. Lewis describes it this way: "You don't have a soul. You are a soul. You have a body."

We neglect this part of our lives at our own peril, becoming preoccupied with our physical bodies or driven by every changing emotional wind.

Much of the time we are that jumbled mess I spoke of earlier, and our lives look like what we see through a kaleidoscope, only nowhere near as pretty. But behind those beautiful colors and shapes are hard, sharp, ever-shifting shards of glass—just as it is within each of us. It's a tough place to be, and we seek ways to find balance and to find peace.

Finding that balance—that sweet spot—is a lifelong journey. But it's not an impossible one. Notice the chair in the center of the illustration below. Actually it's a throne, and it's the *key* to our balance and peace.

This is the very center of our lives, the very seat of our being. And it poses a question that is critical for each of us. And each of us, whether we acknowledge it or not, answers this question every day of our lives. *Who sits on that throne?* If we put ourselves there, we're bound for failure. If we're the captain of our ship, the master of our destiny, well…good luck. And if we place another person there, we're headed for disaster as well. We all suffer from the limitations of being human, and we will hurt and disappoint each other—even our friends and loved ones.

Here's where we're constantly playing musical chairs, circling that throne each day, waiting for the music to stop and see who jumps into that seat—who's going to be in charge of our lives. It's usually us, or because of some circumstance or crisis, it could be a friend or loved one. But that will only be temporary. Our desire, our nature is to be in that chair.

But someone else could occupy that throne—the Man from Galilee. He stands patiently waiting for each of us, waiting for us to choose. He knows our hearts, and understands what pastor and author A.W. Tozer said: "Every man lives by faith, the nonbeliever as well as the saint; the one by faith in natural laws and the other by faith in God."

I chose faith in God, the author of our natural laws. With the balance, centeredness, and peace that he brings from his presence on that throne, we're able to handle whatever this brief life throws our way—whether it be physical challenges or emotional turmoil.

Balance. The sweet spot. It's where we were created to live.

Frequently Asked Questions

We help hundreds of people in our clinic with their lipid problems and try to answer a lot of questions. The preceding pages have provided a bunch of information and dealt with many of these questions, but I think it's a good idea to respond here to some of the most frequently asked questions. You might be wondering about some of them yourself.

Q: If I start a statin drug for my cholesterol, will I have to take it for the rest of my life?

It all depends. Many people who are able to lose weight, change their eating patterns, and get adequate exercise may be able to be weaned off their medication. That would be our goal. I'm a firm believer that the less medicine we have to take, the better off we will be. On the other hand, those of us with profound lipid abnormalities or a clear genetic predisposition will probably be taking these drugs forever. There are worse things.

Q: Some guys at work told me Lipitor would affect my love life and make it worse. Is that true?

Depends on how it was to start with. As a rule, erectile dysfunction is not a side effect of statins. We frequently encounter this complaint with several of our blood pressure medicines as well as those used for anxiety and depression.

Q: I work the night shift. When should I take my simvastatin?

The first time I was asked this question, I had to scratch my head. Shift work reverses our normal cortisol fluctuations, turning them upside down. Likewise, I wondered what effect day/night reversal might have on cholesterol metabolism. Remembering that we manufacture cholesterol and LDL during our fasting periods (usually at night), it seemed reasonable that we should be taking our "night-time meds" when we go to bed, whether that be at 10:00 p.m. or 7:00 a.m. That's the conventional wisdom at this point, supported by several experts in this area.

Q: Do you think Jesus's disciples adhered to the Mediterranean Diet?

Actually, no one's ever asked me this, but I'm curious. It might have been more like the Jordan River Diet. Certainly they would have relied on fruits (figs, grapes, pomegranates, dates), whole grains, wine, and fish. But since the life expectancy at that time was estimated to be between thirty and forty years, and since it takes several decades for cardiovascular disease to manifest itself, we'll never know if this diet conferred any significant heart health benefits.

Q: Doc, you told me my cholesterol is high. Can I still eat eggs for breakfast?

Absolutely, just not on a bagel with a piece of ham. The ham would be okay, it's the bagel we have to worry about. Remember, we were wrong about low-cholesterol/low-fat diets as a way to improve cholesterol levels. Or anything for that matter. These diets rely heavily on carbohydrates for our energy and calorie source—something we now know drives our lipids, blood sugar, and blood pressure in the wrong direction. Low carbs along with lean meats—that's where we need to be headed. Do that, and you can eat your eggs.

Q: If I can get my lipids in order, will it reduce my risk for heart disease?

Yes. A mountain of data exists that supports this. In addition, normal lipid levels will help prevent the development of several other significant diseases—peripheral vascular disease, strokes, and pancreatitis among others.

Q: I read somewhere that the newer statin drugs were better than the old ones. Should I switch from my simvastatin?

How are your lipids doing? If you've achieved your target goals, don't mess with success. The bottom line here is that most people can reach those goals with the earlier statins—simvastatin and pravastatin—while saving money. Just remember, though, you'll need those lifestyle changes to *really* see something happen.

Q: A friend recommended a teaspoonful of mustard for nighttime leg cramps. Not sure if the cramps were due to my Lipitor, but I tried the mustard and it helped. Any harm in doing that?

My grandfather, an owner of fishing schooners at the turn of the century (that would be 1900), would frequently say, "Any port in a storm." I would agree. If it works, do it. Mustard's not going to hurt anyone. I've actually recommended this to a half-dozen of my patients, and they've all gotten relief. Go figure.

Q: I'm forty-two—how often should I have my cholesterol checked?

By "cholesterol" I assume we're talking about your lipid profile. If you enjoy good health and don't take any medication for your lipids, once every five years may be enough. If something happens in the meantime— significant weight gain, thyroid disease, new-onset diabetes—it will be prudent to have it checked more often, maybe every year or two. If you're taking a statin or one of the other lipid-lowering drugs, you'll probably want to have those levels checked every year.

Q: My HDL is 40 and I want to get it higher without taking any prescription medicine. Any ideas?

The wisdom has been to increase your level of exercise. Been there, done that, doesn't work. Or at least not for me. Running five miles a day didn't budge it. What really impacted my HDL level—taking it from 42 to 80— was changing to a low-carb diet. I lost weight, my LDL went down, and my HDL skyrocketed. No meds, nothing else, just the elimination of car-bohydrates wherever I could find them.

Q: My cholesterol and LDL are fine, but my triglycerides are over 300. My cousin says that's okay, as long as the other stuff is normal. What do you think?

I think you need to get your medical advice from a different cousin. It's great that your other lipids are normal, but a significantly elevated tri-glyceride level is a risk in and of itself for cardiovascular disease. This would be the time to increase your consumption of fish and add a fish oil supplement.

Q: Speaking of fish oil—I take one capsule every night and my wife tells me my breath smells like sardines. And she complains about the garlic I've been taking too. What am I supposed to do?

First, step back just a little. The garlic is something you can stop taking. There is no solid evidence that it makes much difference with your lipid levels. The fish breath can be helped by freezing those capsules before you take them. I've tried it and it works.

Q: Which is better for me, butter or margarine?

As a lover of butter, it grieves me to say it's going to be margarine. Just be sure it contains mainly unsaturated fats. Some products will mix different things into the blend and promote it as healthy. Stay away from the satu-rated stuff and you'll be fine. Still, a little butter now and then shouldn't be a problem.

Q: Doc, see these white rings around the dark part of my eye? My nephew's studying premed and he tells me that's a sure sign of high cholesterol. Is he right?

No, those rings are called *arcus senilis* and are very common, especially as we grow older. While they are thought to be deposits of fatty material, they don't correlate with any lipid abnormality and they won't affect your vision. That's something your nephew will understand in a couple of years.

Q: But Dr. Lesslie, I don't have time to wait for my nephew to get through med-ical school. How do I go about contacting you with a question or comment?

I'm always happy to receive comments about anything I've written, and I will try to answer any question you may have. The best way to contact me is at http://robertlesslie.com/blog.

58

The Finish Line

Three months had passed, and Lisa and Dave were back in the office. Their labs were attached to their charts, and I studied each of them. This was going to be a better visit.

The door closed behind me and I pulled over the rolling stool.

"So, have you seen your results?"

Lisa nodded and Dave grinned.

"Your nurse showed them to us," he said. "They look pretty good, don't they?"

"They're a lot better," I agreed, thumbing through his wife's record. "Lisa, you've lost five pounds and your triglyceride level is well below normal—128. That's a great number."

"It must be the fish oil you recommended, Dr. Lesslie. We've stayed with the Mediterranean Diet and we're both exercising. That's the only thing different that I've done."

"Well, it's working, Lisa. All of your other lipids are good, and if that fixes your triglycerides, I'd stick with it."

"Don't worry about that. I've even convinced Dave to start taking fish oil."

I tossed Lisa's chart on the counter and opened his.

"Let's see…you've lost another eight pounds, Dave. Good work there. That's not easy."

"Like I said last time, I feel like I've got fruit and olive oil coming out of my ears, but it looks like it's working. That and the simvastatin we started."

I glanced up at him. "Any problems with it? Leg cramps or muscle pains?"

"Nope, I feel great. Had a little trouble with the niacin you told me to take. It made me flush some, but I take it at night with a baby aspirin and that went away."

"Great."

I held his lab report and went through the numbers again. Dave's total cholesterol had started at 289 and was now 188. His LDL had been dangerously high at 160 and had dropped to 99. And his HDL had gone up from 41 to 50.

"These are all good levels, Dave. And your triglycerides continue to be normal. Good work."

"So, we just continue what we're doing?" He glanced at his wife and back to me.

"That's right. If you're doing fine with these medicines and your lifestyle changes, I'd say just keep at it. We won't need to see you again for a year."

I stood up, stepped toward the door, and stopped. Dave's chart was almost closed when I saw it.

"Hmm..."

"What is it, Doc? What's the matter?" Dave asked.

"It's your blood pressure. We were focused on your lipids, and I didn't notice it. It's a little high—not dangerously so, but we'll need to do something about it."

"Let me guess—another risk factor."

He was right, but we would be able to do something about it.

59

Putting It All Together

If you have a problem with your lipids, now's the time to start doing something about it. And if you just want to improve your overall health, there's no time like the present.

We've looked at a lot of different ideas and topics, and considered multiple ways to get your lipids in line. Let's go through a process that has helped many of my patients make sense of all the things we've talked about. I've listed the key chapters where you'll be able to find more information about each topic.

1. First, you've *got* to know your numbers. These are simple blood tests that will give your physician the information he or she needs to help direct you to the right treatments. What you don't know can hurt you.

> Chapter 3, "Clyde Anderson"
> Chapter 20, "The Eyes Have It"
> Chapter 27, "Tick…Tick…Tick"
> Chapter 39, "Procrastination"
> Chapter 52, "Too Soon"

2. Understand what the numbers mean.

> Chapter 7, "What Exactly Are We Talking About?"
> Chapter 8, "Now About Your Numbers…"

Chapter 14, "Your Total Cholesterol"
Chapter 18, "HDL"
Chapter 24, "LDL"
Chapter 45, "The Other Stuff"

3. Be convinced this is important, because it is. It's all about motivation, and this will happen when we know what's at stake.

Chapter 2, "What *Is* the Big Deal?"
Chapter 4, "What's the Risk?"
Chapter 17, "The Dreaded Syndrome X"

4. Commit yourself to lifestyle changes. This is the bedrock of making improvements with your lipids and improving your health.

- Weight—know your body mass index (BMI). Establish a reasonable goal and work to achieve it.

- Exercise

  Chapter 19, "Get Moving"

- Diet

  Chapter 9, "What Diet Is Best for Me?"
  Chapter 11, "The Low-Carb Approach"
  Chapter 13, "A Couple of Diet Options"
  Chapter 15, "Please Pass the Cardboard: The Importance of Fiber"
  Chapter 16, "Where's the Beef?"
  Chapter 25, "It's Okay to Go a Little Nuts"
  Chapter 53, "Your Momma Was Right: Eat Your Fruits and Vegetables"

- Drinking enough water

  Chapter 23, Water Is Our Friend"

- Adequate Sleep

  Chapter 22, "How'd Ya Sleep Last Night?"

5. Reduce your stress level.

> Chapter 21, "You Just Need to Calm Down"

6. Consider trying some proven supplements.

> Chapter 35, "Niacin"
> Chapter 37, "The Buzz About Antioxidants"
> Chapter 49, "Somethin's Fishy Around Here"
> Chapter 51, "Vitamin D and Your Heart"

7. If lifestyle changes don't get the job done and you need medication, work closely with your physician to find the right one(s). Ask the hard questions:

- "What's the best medication for my particular problem?"
- "What's the upside of this medicine? And the downside?"
- "What should I be looking out for?"

8. Become familiar with our lipid-lowering medications.

> Chapter 30, "The Other Benefits of Statins"
> Chapter 31, "Statins: The Downside"
> Chapter 34, "What Are Some of the Other Drugs?"

9. Don't jump on the latest and greatest bandwagon. Weigh the evidence carefully before modifying your treatment plan.

> Chapter 46, "Biostatistics"
> Chapter 47, "A Guide to the Latest Studies"
> Chapter 48, "When Liars Figure"

10. Monitor your progress regularly. Keep a record of your weight and your lab studies, and see your physician often enough.

11. With your health, as with everything in your life, find balance.

> Chapter 56, "It's All About Balance"

12. Trust in your efforts and believe in your success.

I have learned the secret of being content
in any and every situation,
whether well fed or hungry,
whether living in plenty or in want.
I can do all this through him
who gives me strength.
Philippians 4:12-13

You Gotta Know Your Numbers

You gotta know your numbers. Period.

> "Wisdom is the right use of knowledge."
> Charles Spurgeon (1834–1892)

About the Author

Bestselling author Dr. Robert Lesslie is a physician with more than 30 years of experience working in or directing fast-paced, intense ER environments. He is now the co-owner and medical director of two urgent-care facilities. He has written *Notes from a Doctor's Pocket, Angels on the Night Shift, Angels and Heroes, Angels on Call, Miracles in the ER,* and *Angels in the ER* (over 200,000 sold) as well as newspaper and magazine columns and human-interest stories. He and his wife, Barbara, live in South Carolina.

You can contact Dr. Lesslie through his blog at http://robert lesslie.com/blog.

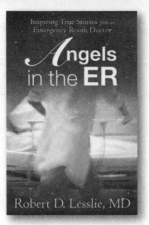

Angels in the ER
Inspiring True Stories from an Emergency Room Doctor

Twenty-five years in the ER could become a résumé for despair, but for bestselling author Dr. Robert D. Lesslie it's a foundation for inspiring stories of everyday "angels"—friends, nurses, doctors, patients, even strangers who offer love, help, and support in the midst of trouble.

"The ER is a difficult and challenging place to be. Yet the same pressures and stresses that make this place so challenging also provide an opportunity to experience some of life's greatest wonders and mysteries."

Dr. Lesslie illuminates messages of hope while sharing fast-paced, captivating stories about

- discovering lessons from the ER frontline
- watching everyday miracles unfold
- holding on to faith during tragedy and triumph
- embracing the healing balm of hope

If you enjoy true stories of the wonders of the human spirit, this immensely popular book is a reminder that hope can turn emergencies into opportunities and trials into demonstrations of God's grace.

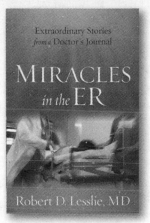

Miracles in the ER
Extraordinary Stories from a Doctor's Journal

You've heard about them. Extraordinary…unexplainable…seemingly miraculous true stories that couldn't have happened—but did. Real-life stories of life changes, answered prayers, inner and outer healing where they appeared impossible.

Again and again, bestselling author Dr. Robert Lesslie has encountered such *Miracles in the ER* during his decades of experience in emergency medicine. In these vignettes—all true stories—Dr. Lesslie chronicles miracles of…

- physical healing
- joy and forgiveness
- restored relationships
- time granted and spent
- angels—human and otherwise

These touching, dramatic, thought-provoking snapshots of life will grace you with hope and prompt you to look more closely for the miracle stories around you that so often go unseen and untold.

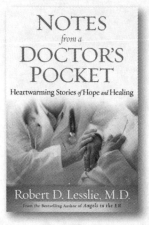

Notes from a Doctor's Pocket
Heartwarming Stories of Hope and Healing

These *Notes from a Doctor's Pocket* come from the decades of ER experience of bestselling author Dr. Robert Lesslie, whose routine faced him with times of grief or pain, relief or delight, life or death. Such everyday happenings and encounters gave rise to these vignettes—in which you will meet up with the characters, coincidences, and complications common to the emergency room:

- characters like Freddy, who literally shoots himself in the foot

- coincidences like finally having the chance to hear what patients say to each other when doctors and nurses aren't in the room

- complications such as dealing with parents who buy lottery tickets and alcohol instead of medicine for their little boy

These heart-tugging, heart-lifting slices of life will prompt you to search for opportunities to give the comfort of a touch, the grace of a kind word, or a prayer that brings hope and healing.